D1296055

THE
Self-Care
IN
Health Care
REVOLUTION

**Learn-One, Teach-One Resources
for Out-of-the-Box Nursing**

DONNA NAUMANN, RN, FNP-BC, HC

The Self-Care in Healthcare Revolution
Learn-One, Teach-One Resources for Out-of-the-Box Nursing
Donna Naumann, RN, FNP-BC, HC
Smile Divine Joy

Published by Smile Divine Joy, O'Fallon, MO
Copyright ©2021 Donna Naumann, RN, FNP-BC, HC
All rights reserved.

Cover and Interior design: Davis Creative, DavisCreative.com

Library of Congress Cataloging-in-Publication Data
Library of Congress Control Number: 2021907080
The Self-Care in Healthcare Revolution
Learn-One, Teach-One Resources for Out-of-the-Box Nursing
Donna Naumann, RN, FNP-BC, HC
ISBN: 978-1-7368835-0-1 (paperback)
 978-1-7368835-1-8 (ebook)
Subject headings:

1. MED004000 MEDICAL / Alternative & Complementary Medicine
    2. MED024000   MEDICAL / Education & Training 3. MED058140   MEDICAL / Nursing / Nurse & Patient

2021

ATTENTION CORPORATIONS, UNIVERSITIES, COLLEGES AND PROFESSIONAL ORGANIZATIONS: Quantity discounts are available on bulk purchases of this book for educational, gift purposes, or as premiums for increasing magazine subscriptions or renewals. Special books or book excerpts can also be created to fit specific needs. For information, please contact Smile Divine Joy, donnanaumann@gmail.com.

Dedication

I dedicate this book to the countless patients I have had the pleasure of serving over the years. You have no idea just how much you have impacted who I am as a teacher, a friend, a counselor, a provider, an empathic individual. Over the years, your stories are what have lifted me to do this work. I felt your pains and traumas and wanted to help you feel better, live better, be better. Our time together inspired this book. I would have no book without you. During our time together, my thoughts were brewing and stories were forming. Something in your stories, pains, fears, and tears spurred me to want to do more. You awakened my own fears and pains that I needed to work on. Thank you so much. I love each and every one of you.

Dedication goes out to all of my lifetimes, all of my ancestors, and all of my inner guidance.

Table of Contents

Acknowledgments

First and foremost, I want to thank my husband, who always lets me dream and believes in me no matter what. Without him, nothing would be possible. He supported my dream of writing a book and never complained about the countless hours I spent writing. I learned love and patience from him, and writing a book needs both of those things. I love you, Ken! You make my heart sing.

To my children, I thank you because you have always accepted my weirdness and supported me in ways you don't even know. Thank you for being great role models to me over the years, teaching me to love, to cherish the moments, to be present. The stepping stones of being a parent taught me so much. I love you Sadie, Jaime, and David. In you, I see the light of love and God.

To my mother, who instilled in me the love of reading and going to the library. Thank you, Mother, for all of your support. You encouraged me to become a critical thinker and allowed me the freedom to explore my world.

Thank you to my sister Debbie, who walked me to the library when I was too young to go alone, and who always took care of me as her little sister. To my other sisters, Dawn and Patty, and my brothers, Mike and Vic—you play an integral role in who I am as a person. Thank you for being who you are and for being a part of my life story.

To my father, who is looking down from heaven, I realize your life was my gift. Without you and my mother, I would not be! You taught me to want to love deeply and be committed to my relationships. Thank you!

For their help writing the book, I want to love on my first editor who initiated the dream, Nancy Erickson. Without her, I would have never had a starting point. Then, I was inspired by Gina Nicole to meet Cathy Davis, who rebirthed my dream. I was able to begin dreaming up the content. Pam Wilson gave me the kick start, and Cheryl Oliver helped me round the bases to home. Cheryl, thank you so much for your enthusiasm and encouragement. It was quite the undertaking, and you made it so easy. I also would like to mention Allison Barnett for helping me write the chapter on stories. What a great job she did. Each and every one of you has been an integral part of my book.

A special shout out to Gina Nicole, Kristen Brokaw, Barbara Goodman Siegel, Stacey O'Byrne, Dawn Ferguson, Stacy Fidler, and Tom Hill. All of these coaches helped me recognize that I needed to bring my spirit into the world. They are always stimulating me to level up, try harder, become inspired, and to inspire and encourage others. I am grateful for the light you shine in this world.

I would like to thank my first physician mentor, Dr. Eckert. You gave me a job that turned into a life of passion and commitment. I learned how to take care of patients, how to go the extra mile, how to become the provider I am today. Your compassion shines through to everyone who knows you. Thank you for always making me laugh and feel like what I was doing really mattered.

Toastmasters taught me to speak up and learn how to be creative in writing. I love you, Toastmaster members, for believing in me.

I had teachers who inspired me, and even though I cannot remember their names, I can see their faces. Thank you to all the teachers in the world! You have no idea whose lives you will impact later in life. It is a hard job, and you do it with so much love.

To God, who is always working inside of me so I can be a better person, **believe in who I am and let my spirit soar in the universe—thank you for putting the people** I needed in my life to help me along the way. Also, I must acknowledge how grateful I am and how much I appreciate the universe, the trees, the sun, the wind, the air, the ocean, the energy! While writing, I looked inward, outward and upward for insight and guidance to find the right words so I could share my stories.

To everyone, thank you for being my angels.

FEARLESSLY PROTECT YOUR LIGHT

There is no greater fight in our life.
We cannot know what we do does matter
Because our heads are full of busy ol' chatter.
We came here to serve and indeed that's what we do.
It can make us happy or it can make us blue.
But what if we learned a new trade or two?
Wouldn't it change our point of view?
Is it possible to become someone better?
How about if we became a new trend setter?
I know that I have a light to shine all around.
I want you to have it so you'll get the crown.
We can do so much more together.
If we help each other, we will all get better.
Don't give up, change is just up ahead.
If we work on ourselves, it can do nothing but spread.
I love you all, you'll never know why
Until you begin to give this stuff a try.
My heart goes out to all of you
In the greatest of fashion of deep gratitude.
Thank you for taking your precious time to learn with
  me.
The truth and the nature of who you can be will certainly
  set you free.

-Donna C. Naumann

Preface

My first experience of 'seeing' a patient was my great-grandmother, Mae Hall. She looked old to me through my youthful eyes of 9. I remember her shuffling across the foyer of my Grandma Jobs' resort, steering toward the nearest bathroom as she leaked across the floor. I could hear my Grandma Jobs scolding her for making a mess and leaving her to have to clean it up. I remember feeling so sad for her. She knew that she was peeing on herself, but truly couldn't stop it. My heart went out to her as I somehow intuitively knew how she felt.

As the years passed, Great-Grandma Hall stopped walking. I remember my Aunt Ada caring for her like she was her own mother. When Great-Grandma Hall couldn't get up anymore, Aunt Ada would give her a bath in bed. She would brush her hair, wash her face, change her bedding, and talk to her in a sweet loving voice. Aunt Ada was clueless to the lessons she was teaching me about becoming an empathetic caregiver, but I got such a powerful sense of her love and compassion. It was easy to see she was making a difference. In my heart, I knew I wanted to make a difference, just like her.

My first real job at 16 years old was for the Visiting Nurse Association. It was my entry into the field of health care. That job influenced me to apply for nursing school. Excitedly, I began my journey of loving on people. I loved them all and wanted to bring everyone hope. If they were crabby, I got them more water and lingered around to figure out what was wrong. If they cried, I held their hand. If they died,

I prayed feverishly over them. The love just came out of me without even trying. This is when you know you are living your purpose.

That love of people started me on a quest to discover new ways to help patients get better. Even when patients were told there was nothing else to be done, I searched for health options outside the box. This guided me toward all of the techniques I have included in this book.

To test these out-of-the-box modalities, I became my first patient. I worked on myself before teaching other people. I began to see my practice grow stronger. Patients who were initially hesitant about seeing me as a nurse practitioner became a permanent part of my schedule. They were comfortable asking me all kinds of questions about their health. I learned that they wanted to be heard and understood. Don't we all?

After completing nursing school, I started working my way through functional medicine, nutrition, Reiki, Pranic Healing, Hypnotherapy, and neuro-linguistic programming. I just kept absorbing information, trying things out, and sharing with patients.

God knows I needed the healing as much as they did. I figured out that if I learned one thing and taught that one thing to another, it deepened my own understanding. The notion of 'teach one, learn one' has been around for years; there always have been teachers and students. For me, it was both selfish, in that I healed myself, and selfless, as I gave lovingly to others. I refer to it as being a *healthpreneur*—an entrepreneur of healing endeavors.

I was motivated by the stories of patients healing through the processes I learned and taught. They compelled me to combine the various resources and techniques that proved so beneficial into this guide for anyone providing care in the healing arts.

I hope my stories will encourage you to want to do more, too. This isn't just for providers. We all need to be our loving selves and stand in our own light. We can start by sorting through the choices offered here. I invite each of you to pick and choose what seems right for you, your patients, and your practice. Implement them and you will see amazing results, just like I did.

I built a whole practice using these techniques. I had patients that wanted to see me instead of the doctor because I was in tune with who they were and what they needed.

It's exciting to learn new things, especially things that I can use to help other people heal. It's amazing to have tools that really work to help other people!

As I write this, we are in the midst of a pandemic that is affecting our health care systems, our own lives and families, and the way we live. So much of what we took for granted has been redirected to address the necessary safety protocols for work, school, and family gatherings. These are trying times indeed, which means we MUST work harder and smarter on our connections.

That just means we have to tool up. And that is the reason for writing this book: to help each of us become not just better providers of care, but better communicators and connectors, and better at our own self-care.

We need each other. And since it's our calling to work and connect with people, it's time that we learn how to do that through proven strategies. One of the most powerful healing tools we have is how we communicate. How we listen and question. I can't say enough about the importance of neuro-linguistic programming and motivational interviewing to open patients up, help them tell their story, and, finally, get to the root of their problems.

This is a time when we are all challenged to learn who we are within our own selves and the light of God. We have energy sources within us that never were and never will be taught in school, but by calling upon that energy, we can connect with patients more quickly and on a higher level than ever before. This book addresses the depression, anger and despair that are surfacing in abundance during this uncertain time. Applying learned techniques of being present, asking questions, and listening will help other people feel understood and loved, which in turn, helps *us* feel understood and loved. It's a win-win for all involved.

My challenge is for each of us to take one chapter of this book and work on it for a month. Observe, journal, experience the changes in yourselves, and then share that change with others.

My promise is that it is impossible to stay the same when you begin to learn a new way. If we practice once a day to think and be another way, then eventually that will become our natural way. It's about learning with intention.

Please know that what we do as intentional, compassionate providers of care matters now more than ever before. We are spiritual beings having a physical experience. What each of us does affects another, individually and collectively, in some small way, even if we aren't overtly aware of it.

Use this book as a resource guide to build awareness, focus intention and invest in yourself as a healer at a time when the world is in dire need of healing. Open the book. Let's get started!

Chapter One

The Calling

The groundwork for all happiness is good health.
-Leigh Hunt

The clear night sky offers a beautiful array of shining white stars. I stare boldly into the full moon, wondering what kind of patients I will take care of tonight. I am on the 18th floor of Barnes-Jewish Hospital in St. Louis, Missouri, looking out over Forest Park on one side and the parking garage on the other. All of the rooms are filled with patients waiting to be tucked in for the night.

After finishing my report, I walk into my first patient's room to get her blood pressure, check her pulse, look at her IV site and fluid levels, and check her kidney transplant site. She just received her new kidney today, and she's been having a slow start of urine. I ask her how she is feeling. As she turns to look at me, I see the tears rolling down her cheeks. I can sense the fear in her eyes. She's had a tough day.

She starts to cry harder and her voice quivers out, "My kidney wasn't putting out a lot of urine today. What if I have to go back on dialysis?" she asks. "I just can't go back on dialysis. I hate it!"

I look down at my assessment sheet and all of the questions I have to address. I set the paperwork down; it will have to wait. I sit on the side of her bed, take her hand and let her cry for a few minutes. When she finishes, I tell her she is going to be fine. This kidney just needs a little jump start and some fluids. She relaxes some, and I smile at her as I reassure her that she had a very successful surgery, and she is going to have a great life with her new kidney. Today, I answered my calling, the first of many that I will experience over the years to come.

The Hierarchy of Health Care

I started my nursing training in 1983. It was a time when nurses wore white caps, white dresses, white tights, and white shoes. We were there to follow orders, assist patients, provide medications, and give baths.

I remember as a student, I was sitting at the nursing station writing my notes when a doctor walked up. All of the chairs in the nursing station were taken. I could see my nursing instructor, who was sitting across the aisle, give me my mother's raised-eyebrow look that said, "Get up." I picked up my chart and gave him my seat. In those days, it was expected that when the doctor showed up, as a nurse, you served him, too.

In the early days, I was under the doctor giving my seat up and in the later years, I was building my own nurse practitioner practice. Wow! Changing times indeed. I have built a nurse practitioner-owned practice in a state where it is rarely seen. Today, nurses are trained to question orders and, as nurse practitioners, to write them. As a group, nurses have become stronger and more vocal about what they need and what patients need. This gives nurses a great opportunity to make positive changes in health care. We are better able to assess patients, defend them, and advocate for them.

At the same time, we face a complicated health care system that is bent on putting money before lives. We have created multiple layers of providers; patients are ranked by acuity levels; and coordinators come by and question the discharge plans.

Everyone now defers to the complicated electronic medical record (EMR) to tell us how to care for our patients and use check boxes to get paid. The insurance companies are dictating our patient care and our rights to provide quality care. The backbone of nursing care—

empathy—is getting pushed to the backseat by the new paradigm of electronically calculated health care.

Electronically Calculated Health Care

When I worked in a hospital in 1986, our focus was on patient care. Charting was minimal and required anywhere from 30 to 60 minutes a shift. The rest of my 12-hour shift was spent with the patients at their bedside. I would give them their medications, bathe them, make their beds, do their assessments, help them with meals, transfer them to the chair, and do their respiratory and IV care. This intimate approach to nursing is a thing of the past.

Studies are emerging on patient care that predict nurses will spend less and less time at the patient's bedside. According to an employee study at Barnes-Jewish Hospital in St. Louis, nurses spend 4 hours of their 12-hour shift charting—that's one-third of their day spent documenting care instead of providing it.[1]

Another study showed that there are three subcategories that account for most of nursing practice time. One is documentation (35.3%; 147.5 minutes), the second is medication administration (17.2%; 72 minutes), and the third is care coordination (20.6%; 86 minutes). Patient care activities accounted for approximately 19.3% (81 minutes) of nursing practice time, leaving 7.2% (31 minutes) of nursing practice time for patient assessment and reading of vital signs. The system is trying to steal our patient care connection by having us jump through so many documentation hoops.

This bothers me. Not that accurate documentation isn't important. It is. But many decision makers in health care seem to have lost sight of the total picture involved in healing. The patients have just become a number in a financial reimbursement war.

I decided to write this book because I was experiencing separation from my core ideas and values as a nurse. The insurance companies, pharmaceutical companies, physicians, and electronics medical records all were overpowering my values as a nurse to provide exceptional care. As a nurse, how I should care for patients is directed by simple strokes on the keys of a computer. I follow the care plans set up by computer analysis. Insurance companies deny my testing, refuse to cover medications that the patients need, will not cover home health to monitor patients who are having issues, and even refuse admissions to the hospital. How is that okay?

I am committed to protecting our rights to give patient care, honor our beliefs in empathy, encourage patients at the bedside, and be present with them when they are in the room. It saddens me when I hear patients say, "that doctor (or nurse) didn't listen to me." Patients feel that the provider is in and out, and sometimes they are. I don't want to be a number, and I don't want to give care in a time crunch.

Teaching and Training Nurses

It is time to focus on what we teach in nursing schools to ensure nurses and patients are empowered. Our jobs as nurses cannot be all about medications, IV bags, CT scans, and testing. Nursing was derived to assist patients in developing self-care, to educate patients, and to help ease their pain.

It's time for nursing schools to embrace new tools that will help students learn about different modalities of healing. Nursing educators need to remember that most nurses will not stay in the hospital setting. Students need to consider the multiple layers of healing for themselves, as well as their patients.

I was invited to speak to students at Goldfarb School of Nursing at Barnes-Jewish College. I was thrilled to have the opportunity to talk to the future nurses of the world and introduce them to the many modalities of healing that I have learned over the years. I shared what I saw as the weaknesses in Western medicine: we stop helping patients after the IV is hung, the blood sugars normalize, or their chemotherapy is completed.

My question for them was, "What is next for nurses and patients today?" I introduced the students to all that I have learned in my quest for healing. I talked about food as medicine, food allergies, gut dysfunction, healing essential oils, Ho'oponopono, meditation, Heart-Math breathing, chakra energy, and vitamin supplements. I was so excited to share with the students all of the possibilities of helping and healing people besides drugs. I finished the presentation psyched and was so proud of myself.

How is it then that when I finished my presentation, the instructor said to me, "That was interesting! That was not what I was expecting." I could feel the sarcasm roll off her lips.

I realized that she had expected me to talk about my role as a family nurse practitioner and owner of a family medical practice, not weave in alternative healing modalities. The instructor would have been content presenting the story of the modern-day nurse practitioner being utilized as a provider but paid like a nurse. I shook my head.

I believe our role is about helping people realize that no one is coming to heal them. They have to work at it and participate in their own healing journey if they really want to get better. They need to learn that there are many self-healing techniques that can be utilized, and there are studies that support their effectiveness. It is time for us, as nurses, to step up our game.

Our ideas of treating disease must change if healing and health are going to merge. I wanted to yell at the teacher and say, "Get out of your box!" Instead, I left feeling guilty for not giving the students the information the teacher had expected. Then I beat myself up for being insecure about what I believe is really important as a nurse. Finally, instead of feeling bad about what I said, I made a vow to spread this energy to anyone that would listen.

Our Calling

My mission is to pass on the gifts of patient care and self-care to nurses and patients. We cannot let the current trends in health care dismiss the patients while causing burnout among caregivers, nurses, and providers. We have to come up with new ideas and solutions to help providers (and caregivers) feel what they do really does matter.

We can't look over our shoulders. No one is coming to spread the word about alternative methods of care. Nurses, it starts with us! It is time for us to learn other ways to help ourselves and others heal. It's all out there! Let's explore it together. Need the science behind it? It is all there too, if we only look. This is our calling. This book is a starting point!

Chapter Two

The Amazing Heart

I suspect it is hard to love a nurse. We get up early and don't have time to drink coffee over the newspaper. We come home late and are too tired to cook. We miss weekend events, holidays, birthdays. We don't get too excited over your minor "boo-boo." We have seen far worse. We don't want to talk when we come home. We have talked all day. We don't want to move when we come home. We have moved all day. It may seem that we have left all our caring, our heart, and our love at work, then have come home to you empty, but our love tank is completely full, just our energy is waning. We don't tell you that many times at work we are mired by anxiety, we are scared. Scared we are missing something. Scared we will let our patient down or worse.

–Maureen Collins Pelletier, RN

Maureen Collins Pelletier is a nurse who cares about nurses, nursing, patients and healing. Her words remind me of how much love we have for our patients. Then, too, we must learn to replenish our own hearts. That is the only way we can go on to the next one who needs us, and to be there for ourselves and our families. It is universal that we give too much and get too little. This is why it is essential for nurses to have the knowledge and skills to easily replenish themselves anytime by simply practicing the techniques in this book. The first step is in understanding the heart and learning how to fill it with love. The second step is to teach others to do the same.

Nurse Judy

Judy was working the night shift in the Cardiac Cath lab. Her main job was to assist the doctors doing heart procedures to look for blockage in the vessels of the heart. It was the doctor's job to identify and clear any blockages before people had a heart attack and died. On this night, they received a call about a 50-year-old male in the emergency room who was having chest pain and needed a cardiac cath procedure stat.

Judy began to quickly prepare the cath lab. Before she could finish her prep work, she got a second call from the emergency room to cancel the procedure. The patient had decided to leave against medical advice when his chest pain resolved. Within an hour, Judy got yet another call from the emergency room.

The man was in an ambulance on his way back to the hospital, and they were going to send him straight to the cardiac cath lab. His wife was with him. By the time he was prepped and ready for his catheter procedure, his pain once again had resolved. He asked if he could make a quick call to his daughter, Elaine. He told her he loved her and assured her that he was fine and hung up. Within minutes of hanging up the phone, the squeezing chest pain came back with a vengeance. Within seconds, he was unconscious and pulseless.

Everyone in the cath lab was frantically doing everything they could to save his life, pushing IV drugs, CPR, shocking his heart with the defibrillator, but his heart would not respond. The minutes ticked by, but still no heartbeat. After 45 minutes, he was pronounced dead despite all of the great medical care that was given that night.

Hearing the words that her husband had been pronounced dead, his wife was struck by shock of a different kind—disbelief. She became hysterical, sobbing loudly, and had no family there to console her.

This is when Judy took off her cardiac procedure hat and put on her compassionate nursing hat. She walked over to the woman and silently hugged her. The wife dropped her head onto Judy's chest and wept, clinging to her for dear life. Judy was sharing the only thing she could in a crisis like this: a compassionate hug, soothing words, and the voice of empathy. In that moment, Judy could feel tears in her own eyes as she understood that deep feeling of loss. This moment was a great reminder for her about why she became a nurse. It's about being with someone and helping them survive a devastating experience. On her way home, Judy thought about the night, feeling deep compassion and a great sense of loss.

*****

It is an honor to include Judy's story—one of millions like it—in this book about hope and heart, about nurses and nursing. That wife will never forget Judy, and Judy will never forget her, either.

Those who have accepted nursing as their calling do so with an understanding that there will be difficult times. It helps knowing that inside each of us is a longing to be held, helped and to be helpful. That is the true beauty of being a nurse.

Heart Impressions

At the core of every nurse is an ability to use empathy to help our patients feel love, acceptance and understanding. It is the ability to sense the things people need because they need the same things we do. We make a lasting impression on people's lives whether we realize it or not.

We are all connected to each other. We all have lived knowing love, having love and giving love. Maybe we've broken someone's heart, or someone has broken our heart. I don't think anyone gets out of this lifetime without having lived through a broken heart. That feeling that the world has ended and may never be the same again can be both brutal and beautiful because it creates empathy inside each of us, that ability to feel the pain of another. This is the center of what we do as nurses. We live from the heart, and by living from the heart, we are able to touch others' lives and support them on their healing journey.

The Amazing Heart

The heart has an amazing ability to beat about 120,000 times a day, sending 2,000 gallons of blood surging through 60,000 miles of blood vessels, feeding all of the organs and tissues. The workings of the heart are faster than the speed of light. The heart's electrical field is approximately 60 times greater in amplitude than the brain and 100 times greater in strength. This magnetic field runs through our body and then surrounds us, extending out 3 feet into our universe. We can use this amazing capacity and power to make a difference—simply by holding someone's hand or standing within their 3-foot energy field. Producing empathy and love becomes easy when you understand the far-reaching parameters of the heart. You can touch anyone energetically, empathetically and lovingly.

Using the Heart to Make a Difference

I first heard Leo Buscaglia, Ph.D., speak on Nine PBS television. I was going through a rough breakup and feeling down. As I watched, tears began to slide down my cheeks. I listened to him express his passion about love and how we all need so much of it. I just sat there weeping and nodding my head in agreement. I definitely felt it was lacking in my life. As I listened, I learned that I am responsible to be love for others and for myself. For myself? I never really thought about loving myself. I always thought of love as something you got from someone else. I listened as he spoke directly to my heart, and I fell in love with love. Loving others and myself. His work and videos are passionate and so true to life. I wanted that kind of love in my life.

Leo Buscaglia was very committed to spreading love and teaching love. He started a college class entitled 'Love' and offered it for free. None of the professors or advisors thought that students would sign up for that "silly class," but he did it anyway. The door to his class opened and soon the room was overflowing with students who wanted to learn about love. After that, he invested his life promoting love as the path of living in fullness. He was born a teacher, and he created his legacy as Dr. Love. Love is easy, according to Leo Buscaglia. In his book, he states: " … return to touching each other, to holding each other, to smiling at each other, to thinking about each other, to caring about each other. Lastly, the loving individual is one who hasn't forgotten his own needs." (pg. 32 *Living, Loving & Learning*)

I think nurses have a lot of love along with the unique opportunity to inject small doses in their patients every day. We have a powerful ability to patch broken hearts—our own, our patients and our loved ones. Nurses really do change the world with simple acts of kindness, reflecting the true nature of healing and being present with our patients in the middle of a crisis. We fill in huge, aching gaps of loneliness with love. Caring for our patients is what makes their stay in the hospital bearable. It's up to us to plant the seeds of love and watch the healing grow.

The Greatest Salesman in the World

I was introduced to the work of Og Mandino in his book, *The Greatest Salesman In the World*. I spent months reading and rereading the most important scrolls of life. He writes that one of the greatest gifts of a salesman is to love.

Here is a small insert from his second scroll:

> *"But how will I react to the actions of others? With love.*
> *For just as love is my weapon to open the hearts of men,*
> *love is also my shield to repulse the arrows of hate and*
> *the spears of anger. Adversity and discouragement will*
> *beat against my new shield and become as the softest of*

rains. My shield will protect me in the marketplace and sustain me when I am alone. It will uplift me in moments of despair, yet it will calm me in time of exultation. It will become stronger and more protective with use until one day I will walk unencumbered among all manners of men and, when I do, my name will be raised high on the pyramid of life.

"I will greet this day with love in my heart.

"And how will I confront each whom I meet? In only one way. In silence and to myself I will address him and say I Love You. Though spoken in silence these words will shine in my eyes, unwrinkle my brow, bring a smile to my lips, and echo in my voice; and his heart will be opened. And who is there who will say nay to my goods when his heart feels my love?"

After reciting this scroll out loud twice a day for a whole month, I decided that, in my own way, I am a salesman selling love and hope to patients. I decided to implement my own technique at work to see what happened. Here's my simple technique:

1. Open the door to the patient's room.
2. Establish eye contact.
3. Concentrate, and
4. Nonverbally communicate "I love you."

Over time I realized this simple technique was having profound effects on the patients and the practice. I found that I was able to really connect with them. I apply this eye contact of "I love you" to everyone I meet. The results are amazing.

Interestingly, patients often will say, "When you do that thing, I feel so much better." They do not know what that 'thing' is, but I do. I have found if you meet people with an open heart, they will know that you are genuinely there for them. A small, simple act of an intentional "I love you," which costs nothing, truly will alter our interactions and connections for a lifetime.

Nurses who really want to experience the joy of nursing and helping people heal can go a long way by sharing their own silent words of love and extending a warm hand to everyone. In return, we receive love back. We actually are fortunate that we are in a profession that sees people at their worst, because we have the opportunity to give them compassion and love. There is no greater gift.

Heart Hug

I always am striving to feel connected and to be loved. I decided to do a Toastmaster speech competition titled Love, and one of the things I researched about connecting to love was hugging. Hugging is a unique gift. When we hug someone, we create a natural *feel-good* chemical called oxytocin. According to psychotherapist Virginia Satir, we need 12 hugs a day. I thought I was lacking in my number of hugs, so I started to add them at home and at work. During that time, I had teenagers who were not that interested in hugging. I couldn't understand it at all. Some days they would poker up like porcupines.

But that didn't stop me. I went all in, stabbed by their razor-sharp edges, and did it anyway. I really felt that them avoiding hugs must have meant they really needed them. Every morning I went in and did my rounds giving them a big hug, much to their disgust, and my great joy. It felt right for me, and I persisted. It wasn't long until I was adding hugs for my patients as well. Some of them were porcupines too, but when I felt they really needed it, I did it anyway. Most people can feel that they are truly a love connection.

HeartMath

The heart has energy that is picked up on an electrocardiogram, ECG, monitor. It doesn't stop when we turn the monitor off; the beat goes on. Our hearts beat out into the universe where we easily can connect just by being together.

HeartMath[2] uses the ECG to test how clients connect with each other through varying degrees of breath and heart work. It uses science-based technology to reduce stress and anxiety while promoting inner balance and heart intuition.

Applying the motto "living life with heart" to 26 years of research, HeartMath has proven that if we improve emotional well-being and promote healthy lifestyles, we will reduce disease. "Our research suggests the heart also is an access point to a source of wisdom and intelligence that we can call upon to live our lives with more balance, greater creativity and enhanced intuitive capacities. All of these are important for increasing personal effectiveness, improving healthy relationships, and achieving greater fulfillment."

HeartMath techniques are used to synchronize your heart, your breath, and your brain through breathing and visualization. The techniques help relieve stress by staying mindful on the breath and meditating on the heart. When you are living in the heart and through the heart, you actually can heal your spiritual and physical ailments. Healing patients by reducing stress through heart meditation and breathing exercises is long overdue.

The technique:

Step 1. Heart Focus—Focus your attention on the area around your heart, the area in the center of your chest. If you like, place your hand over the center of your chest to help you keep your attention on the heart area.

Step 2. Heart Breathing—Breathe deeply but normally and feel your breath as it is coming in and going out. As you inhale, feel as if your breath is flowing in through your heart, and as you exhale, feel it leaving through your heart. Breathe slightly deeper than normal. Continue breathing with ease until you find a natural inner rhythm that feels good for you.

Step 3. Heart Feeling—As you maintain your heart focus and heart breathing, try to activate a positive feeling. Recall a time when you have felt a feeling of deep love or appreciation. One of the easiest ways to generate a positive, heart-based feeling is to remember a special place you've been or a loved one or pet. This is the most important step. Concentrate and breathe through this. Breathe in love and receive it, then breathe out love and share it.

I am encouraged by this work because the studies are so powerful. Medical schools are now incorporating HeartMath techniques into their curriculum! Heart work is in our future. The research, technologies, and methodologies are permeating our country and are beginning to pulse into the hospital settings. There is a bariatric center in St. Louis where doctors perform gastric bypass and banding for patients. They understand that obesity can be a symptom from stress and anxiety. They know that food can have an emotional attachment for patients. They are committed to helping patients release stress by educating them on breath work and heart work. With their program, when obese patients get stressed, instead of eating, they get relief by using the HeartMath techniques that they learned before surgery. This gives patients a tool that addresses the deeper causes of obesity. Bravo to the providers who have pushed the hospitals to make this happen for their patients.

According to the HeartMath Institute, even being together with others can cause the heart and brain waves to connect and synchronize. Not only do the studies support that slowing the breath down and focusing on the heart can synchronize the heart, the lungs, and the brain waves, it also causes clients to feel calm. The premise is that by simply holding the patient's hand, a nurse can change the patient's brainwaves and synchronize their heart and brain. Imagine if every nurse used these techniques with their patients. (See also Appendix A)

PANDEMIC PROTOCOL NOTE:

During the pandemic, we couldn't touch each other with a beautiful hug, and we must still be thoughtful about being or not being fully vaccinated, but we can always be present with our words, our smiles, and our purposeful eye contact. I would like to offer up also letting the stethoscope linger a little longer over the heart and lungs as a meaningful moment of connection. The pandemic has, of necessity, removed the handshake, the hand holding, the hug, the soft touch on an arm or shoulder, a friendly kiss on the cheek.

Please don't hide behind the mask as a way to escape. Be the provider or nurse that pushes the envelope, using these moments to make others feel warm and cared for. So many of our patients are dying from loneliness right now. They cannot have visitors at the hospital, and families canceled holiday and other celebratory gatherings. You may be the only one that person encounters who can bring them the gift of love. Be that gift. Stay present, share the loving eye contact, and use the moments to just hang in the room for an extra minute.

You can teach yourself the breath work and visualization with the HeartMath techniques. Then teach it to your patients. This is a connection that cannot be broken. There is no touch involved with the HeartMath visualization and breath work, but there is connection on an energy level just by you being present with the patient.

You can improve relationships and communication with your patients using a few simple techniques. What we have lost temporarily makes it even more important to learn and apply these loving tools. Imagine how we can make a difference by sharing a simple touch through eye contact, our gentle voice, and compassion.

Why not allow yourself and your patient to take a moment to actually hug yourselves, that's right, hug yourself, and allow the chemicals of love to explode? We are a species that longs to touch and be together. Without touch, we have lost our feelings of belonging (oxytocin). Give hope to your patients who so desperately need it.

*****

The Perfect Heart

(Original story by Rev. Garry Izzard, rewritten and used with permission.)

A young man was standing in the middle of the town proclaiming that he had the most beautiful heart in the whole valley. A large crowd gathered, and they all admired his heart, for it was perfect. There was not a mark or a flaw in it.

But an old man appeared at the front of the crowd and said, "Your heart is not nearly as beautiful as mine."

The crowd and the young man looked at the old man's heart. It was beating strongly but full of scars. It had places where pieces had been removed and other pieces put in ...

but they didn't fit quite right and there were several jagged edges.

The young man looked at the old man's heart and laughed. "You must be joking," he said. "Compare your heart with mine ... mine is perfect and yours is a mess of scars and tears."

"Yes," said the old man. "Yours is perfect looking ... but I would never trade with you. You see, every scar represents a person to whom I have given my love ... I tear out a piece of my heart and give it to them ... and often they give me a piece of their heart, which fits into the empty place in my heart, but because the pieces aren't exact, I have some rough edges.

"Sometimes I have given pieces of my heart away ... and the other person hasn't returned a piece of his heart to me. These are the empty gouges ... giving love is taking a chance. Although these gouges are painful, they stay open, reminding me of the love I have for these people, too ... and I hope someday they may return and fill the spaces I have waiting. So now do you see what true beauty is?"

The young man stood silently with tears running down his cheeks. He walked up to the old man, reached into his perfect young and beautiful heart, and ripped a piece out. He offered it to the old man.

The old man took his offering, placed it in his heart and then took a piece from his old, scarred heart and placed it in the wound in the young man's heart.

It fit ... but not perfectly, as there were some jagged edges.

The young man looked at his heart, not perfect anymore but more beautiful than ever, since love from the old man's heart flowed into his.

This story reminds me of how Judy connected with the wife after she just lost her husband. I know they exchanged pieces of each other's hearts that day that will keep them connected forever. And I believe the old man must have been a healer.

Each of us has had broken hearts, times when we gave so much and got so little, and other times when we got so much and gave so little. Our hearts are the channels that open and allow us to love one another and care for each other even when we don't know one another. How often a nurse goes in the room and is able to touch the patient's heart and help them see another day.

Chapter Three

Empowering Patients: Motivational Interviewing (MI)

You have two ears and one mouth. Use them in that ratio.
(Motivational Interviewing - Listen to Understand)

Motivational interviewing is a technique that has been taught for years. Although it has been around for a long time, I had never heard of it or used it. Sometimes my conversations were going nowhere and had no punch line. I felt like after seeing the patient, I just left the room without making any connection.

Something was missing.

At lunch one day, Nancy, the Novo Nordisk representative, came in to talk to me about her new medication for diabetes. She was proud of what Novo Nordisk was doing for the diabetic community. She shared that they had a diabetic educator who could come out and teach our office how to handle our diabetic patients better and get better diabetic compliance rates. She asked me if I would like to meet with the diabetic educator. I was happy to have an opportunity to learn more about the program and how it could help the office and the patients.

Weeks later, Connie, the Novo Nordisk educator, came out to teach the staff how to connect with our patients. She first taught us about Motivational Interviewing (MI) and how it can help patients analyze the barriers that prevent them from controlling their diabetes. Connie talked about how to connect with patients, how to discuss health care with them, and which standards of care needed to be addressed at every visit by the medical assistant.

She said things like: "Can you tell me about your procedures when you put a diabetic in the room?" She reflected on the steps the staff was doing right and then asked, "Would it be helpful if I offered up some other strategies that may make it easier for you to obtain information from the patients?" She ended by asking what we thought about the information we learned from her. It was exciting to see the conversation flow and get different perspectives.

As Connie wrapped up, she reminded us not to give too much information each visit because people don't learn when they are overwhelmed with information. Patients only can focus on one thing at a time. Boy, was that going to be a tough one for me.

Motivational Interviewing

I looked more into motivational interviewing and learned that it was established in 1983 by William Miller, professor of psychology, and Stephen Rollnick, a clinical psychologist. They co-authored *Motivational Interviewing: Helping People Change*, which covers their theory of motivational interviewing to promote change in clients. MI involves using specific guided language to promote conversations with people to help them talk themselves into change. MI counselors know that the patients already have arguments for and against their current health care behaviors, which creates a type of ambivalence. MI techniques help clients voice their reasonings for change, even those that are contradictory.

Here are the five questions that MI recommends using to guide our patient conversations regarding changing a current health issue.

Why would you want to make this change?

How might you go about it in order to succeed?

What are the three best reasons for you to do it?

How important is it for you to make this change, and why?

So, what do you think you'll do?

These questions empower patients to engage and feel accepted and understood. Another question I like to add to the list is, "What is stopping you from reaching this goal?" The objective of MI is to help patients self-identify successes and barriers to controlling their diseases. That's a lot. One study by William Miller found that 75% of patients had better outcomes when providers used motivational interviewing. This is compelling evidence that using words with intention and consideration can help others change healthy behaviors.

The change has to start with us, the providers of health care.

I think back to the thousands of other patients I have overwhelmed over the years. Could I have made a larger impact by simply engaging in meaningful conversation?

I've learned that I am able to create a more impactful visit by simply using the proven tools. I think the best MI technique for engaging that I have incorporated is using the acronym OARS.

Using OARS to Engage Patients

- Open-ended questions
- Affirmative statements
- Reflections
- Summarizing statements

Open-Ended Questions

These are conversational questions. They create an open opportunity for the patient to be part of the process. As nurses, we want to learn what the patient needs and wants. Unfortunately, they don't always know what they need and want. Open-ended questions allow patients to share their stories and concerns and help us find out what is at the root of noncompliance. Through careful interviewing, patients are able to self-identify the barriers that are preventing them from making better health care choices.

Here's a great example. My diabetic patient, Michael, misses his insulin and pills several times a week. My usual question is demanding and direct, "Why do you miss your medications, Michael?" This question always makes him feel bad for not doing what he is supposed to do, but that doesn't change his behavior.

After several visits with Michael and still no change, I pulled out my OARS card that I keep in my folding medication pad and changed my approach. I ask him, "Tell me about your medication schedule." He tells me that sometimes he forgets it, or sometimes he takes it to work and then forgets it. He puts his medications in different places. I asked him what he could do to remind himself to take his medications. He thought about it and we went over his morning routine. He gets up with an alarm, brushes his teeth, sometimes he eats and sometimes he doesn't. We discussed putting his meds with his toothpaste and setting an alarm. He responded with, "I never thought about setting my alarm for my medicine. I set an alarm for everything." I reinforced how well he did getting to work on time every day using his alarm. That alarm system will be easy for him. He came up with a solution he had control over and was certain he would be more successful at it. He also left feeling like he was empowered instead of belittled.

Affirmative statements

Affirmative statements enable us to recognize the patients' strengths, successes, and efforts that will help them change. Affirmation helps build collaboration and puts the patient and provider on the same team. For example, when I have a patient who only takes his medications five days out of seven, by pointing out how he is successful five days a week, we then can discuss ways he can use those successful techniques the other two days.

Reflections

When we listen to what the patients tell us, we can learn about their beliefs and barriers. By paraphrasing or repeating back to them what they just said, we encourage them to continue to share. For example, if a patient hears me say, "I understand your frustration with remembering your medications; it can be difficult. I heard you say that you like to take your medications before breakfast. What if you put your medication on the breakfast table? Or can you set a timer for your medications every day to make sure you've taken them?"

Summary Statements

Summary statements allow us to briefly review what has been discussed and draw out the key points that need to be emphasized. This helps the patient have a clear idea of what the visit was about and what decisions were made. For example, regarding testing of blood sugars four times a week, we could ask, "Which days will you choose to test your blood sugars?"

Questions promote great outcomes! The art of asking questions is something we all need to practice. Consider the following questions and decide if they are open-ended questions or closed questions:

- Are you checking your blood sugars at home?
- Can you tell me about your process for checking your blood sugar levels at home?
- Why don't you take your diabetic medication every day?
- What are the barriers to taking your diabetic medication every day?
- If you did take your medicine every day, how do you think it might help you?

Remember, we can start a conversation, or end one, just by how we ask our questions.

- Regard the patient's feelings and readiness for change.
- Don't give advice without asking.
- Allow the patients to offer the change solutions.
- Don't overwhelm the patient with excessive information. Be specific.

As you begin your journey into MI, remember to build in layers one step at a time. Keep a reminder of the one question that you are going to start with taped to your computer or on a sticky note or your badge. Reference it, and after you get good at that one question, add another. I carried my four plastic cards inside my folding medication pad for years, pulling them out for reminders as I needed. It is a joy to talk to patients who can voice their own change plans and know that we helped them become successful by simply changing the questions we asked and how we responded to their change talk.

Chapter Four

The Language of our Bodies: Neuro-linguistic Programing (NLP)

What you do speaks so loudly that I cannot hear what you say.
–Ralph Waldo Emerson

I was finishing up with Bobbie's visit when she took a deep breath and said, "What's the matter with you today?"

I looked at her puzzled. "What do you mean?" She answered, "You are just off today."

"Oh, I'm fine. Anything else you want to discuss today?"

"No. I'm concerned about you. You just aren't acting like yourself." She was so sincere. I was trying to hide my feelings. I looked her in the eye, took a deep breath and explained, "Well, today is Dr. Eckert's last day, and I am feeling very emotional." Then I started to cry. Dr. Eckert and I had been practicing side by side for 15 years. He was like the dad I never had. He always believed in me. I wiped my tears away, and she told me I could handle it and that I would find another great doctor just like him.

I wondered what Bobbie was seeing in me that caused her to think something was wrong. I knew I was upset, but I thought I was holding it all together. I had to stop and analyze who I was being that she would have noticed. What Bobbie noticed was that my facial expression was tight and restrained, my normal upbeat voice was low, and I was staring down at her chart rather than enjoying the "I love

45

you" eye contact I usually had. My arms were crossed as we talked, and I never touched her shoulder. There were clear signs being conveyed by me that I thought I was successfully hiding. Nope.

Nurses take for granted what they are observing in their patients. They naturally see and feel things that are going on in the conversations. Come to find out, the patients are looking at us, too—they are also intuitive. They look to us for confirmation that they are doing okay. When they see something incongruent, they become guarded.

We all have body language that tells a story. I decided that if the patients could tell what was going on with me, then I needed to hone in on the body language skills and use them more purposely.

Now, I love to watch patients' bodies talk. I see their reactions, how they are dressed, their facial expressions, where they are looking, and how they are responding to me. I use all of these observations to help me connect with them. I want thriving patients and a thriving practice. I want to feel I am making a difference by paying attention and being observant.

The Old Way Verses The New Way

I bounce into the room and sit down beside Sue. I smile and quickly notice her red-hot cheeks, tightened lips and a frown she is hurling across the room. She has her arms across her chest as if she were holding a bomb ready to explode.

My instinctive alarm system goes off: "RUN!" Instead, I wait, dumbfounded, as she aims her anger like a spear at my forehead. She stands up and leaves, pushing past me with a grunt. I sit there bewildered about what just happened.

What was it she said about her wait, her bill, her medications being denied?

The rest of the day, I felt drained. All I wanted to do was complain about her to the staff and get them on my side. It was all about validating my feelings. She had definite anger issues. I absorbed her negative energy and allowed it to fester inside of me.

After 25 years of problem solving and energy exhaustion, I knew I was headed for burnout. Then I thought, "There has to be a better way." I didn't want to let yelling, angry patients decide what kind of day I was going to have. And I absolutely refused to keep absorbing other people's negative or sad energy. I was not going to continue to have unsupervised emotions swirling out of control all around me.

I decided to get serious about ways to control my own thoughts and behaviors. If I could learn how to defuse bad situations, and at the same time gain rapport and respect, I could have more days that felt successful instead of feeling stressed. I wanted to feel connected, not exhausted. I wanted to be present, not victimized.

That's when I took a course on neuro-linguistic programming (NLP). I knew immediately it would help me become a better version of myself. I knew it would help me as a wife, mother, and provider. It was a win-win-win.

Now, fast-forward 10 years. Let's revisit how to handle Sue's appointment. Sue is yelling at me. She is talking loudly, fast, and directing her anger at me. She is standing close with arms crossed over her chest. I can feel her heated anger. I respond by paraphrasing her comments and lowering my voice using soft-spoken words. I listen so I can repeat what she is saying to mirror her words and feelings. I match her physical cues, placing my arms where her arms are placed. I slow my breathing. My eye contact is on, silently gleaming "I love you." Her tone lowers; I touch her on her shoulder. The anger has been defused. Tears fill her eyes, and we sit down to engage and explore the source of what is going on with her. She feels like I understand her and that I am listening to her concerns. She matters. I am able to defuse an ugly situation, and we both leave feeling like we were heard. Bad energy evaporated!

Learning to Speak Without Saying a Word

The difference between these scenarios is the incorporation of neuro-linguistic programing (NLP) and verbal and nonverbal communication, things I now integrate into all of my visits.

NLP was developed in the early 1970s by Richard Bandler, a gestalt therapist and computer scientist, working with Dr. John Grinder, a linguist and therapist. They studied the great works of Dr. Milton Erickson, the forerunner of NLP Mirroring and Matching techniques, and the father of modern hypnotherapy.

The combined brilliance of these early leaders and creators of NLP changed *bedside counseling* around the world.

I get excited learning new techniques to help me and my patients. When I stumbled on NLP, I couldn't wait to try it on patients, myself, and my family. I have been studying human behaviors all of my life in some form or fashion. I wanted to learn how to handle my stress and stressful clients. I wanted to be able to dissolve bad situations, and gain rapport and respect. I basically hated absorbing the stress of others, feeling my energy drain away, and spending a whole day feeling exhausted.

Before you read further into this chapter, answer the following questions.

- Do you have a standard greeting for everyone you meet?

- Do you have an organized approach when you introduce yourself to patients?

- Do you use your own special techniques to help patients feel connected and in alignment with your care?

- When you speak, are you predominantly using words that describe feelings, seeing, thinking or hearing?

- Are you interested in connecting with more people, making a bigger impact in your life and in the lives of others?

- Are you curious about why some people have better connections with others and wonder if you can learn it, too?

- Is it important for you to better connect with your boss, coworkers or family?

- Could enhanced customer service contribute to your success?

- Could you feel happier, accepted, and loved by being more sensitive to how you are being?

- Do you believe you can change yourself and your patients' attitudes toward life and wellness through communication?

If you answered yes to all of these questions, you likely are using NLP in your interactions. If you answered no to any/all of these questions, you may want to revisit them after you complete the chapter.

A Fresh Approach

Most people believe that our messages are processed through verbal communication, but it is our nonverbal communication that accelerates connectivity with others. This is definitely good news in an era where face masks have become a standard staple of our attire, hiding our whole face from scrutiny. So, listen up, here's the way around the mask!

Research shows that when we communicate feelings and attitudes, only a small percentage of our overall message comes from the words we use (Mehrabian, 2007).

- 55% of our message comes from body language.

- 38% of our message comes from our tone of voice.
- Only 7% of our message is conveyed by the words we use.

Applying this data opens up a whole new approach to helping patients and clients be heard and understood. Learning to master the verbal and nonverbal patterns that people portray helps us understand patients better. Communication expert Dorothy Leeds states it this way: "No words can convey confidence or lack of it as quickly as body language does, and it takes many brilliant words to change poor impressions made by your nonverbal signals." Wow.

NLP can improve patient-nurse relationships by teaching us how to analyze words, patterns, and behaviors to help communicate better and make a meaningful connection with people. It occurs when we become aware of our dialogue and body language with other people, and therefore are more able to manage our emotions and reactions. The secret is to try to be undetectable while you are being observant. Also realize, nowhere in here have I mentioned that only the lips or smile can portray our communication gifts. So, look outside the face for what is really going on with people. Let's dig deeper.

Establishing Rapport by Mirroring and Matching

One of NLP's power tools involves *mirroring and matching* other people's behavior. This is done by observing their nonverbal communication and applying that to our own nonverbal behavior when we are in a conversation with them.

Examples include:

- They have their feet crossed; you cross your feet.
- They are breathing slow; you slow down your breathing.
- They are leaning forward; you lean slightly forward.

The fact that we are mirroring and matching their nonverbal cues helps them feel like we are similar to them and makes them feel like we understand what they are feeling or saying (mirror, match).

Why? Because people fear being different and accept those who are most like them. Using NLP helps people feel safe, accepted, loved, and understood.

This is true not only in nursing, but in almost every other communication context as well. For example, professor Richard Wiseman carried out a study that involved training waiters using the NLP techniques of mirroring and matching.

The waiters were told to take orders from their tables, with one group of waiters using positive reinforcement, "sure, no problem, great," in response to the customer's order. The other group of waiters was told to mirror their customers by simply repeating the orders back to them. The waiters who used the mirroring technique got a staggering 70% larger average tip than those who used positive reinforcement.

How do we as nurses improve our patient satisfaction scores and increase our impact on patients' health? These are goals worth aspiring to, and the following techniques help us connect with our patients under normal circumstances.

- Mirror their behavior, posture, and arm and leg movements, subtly.
- Mirror their voice volume; is it high or low?
- Mirror their breathing, fast or slow?
- Mirror the speed of their voice.
- Put the right amount of space between you and them; intimate is 0-18 inches, casual/personal/vibrational is 3 feet.

- Mirror their body language; leaning forward or leaning back?

- Observe their behaviors, e.g., open arms or closed arms.

- Touch their arm or shoulder as you do their exam.

- Convey "I love you" silently with eye contact.

- In response to anger, slow down all responses and mirrored movements.

The most beneficial way to establish rapport quickly is to mirror and match during communication. Here are other ways of using the mirroring and matching techniques:

- Crossover Matching—match their behavior. (If they are finger tapping, then do a totally different behavior of your own, like foot tapping.)

- Movements—match their expressions (eyebrows, smile, frown, head up or down) and gestures (arms crossed, legs crossed) without making it too obvious.

- Breathing—this is extremely subtle and powerful. Either match their breathing or crossover match by blinking at the same rate that they breathe.

- Tonality—match the tone, speed, pitch or rhythm of their voice.

Discover Thought Processes

By studying NLP, I learned to listen to clients' vocabulary and discover their predominant thought processes. Thought experience can be feeling, seeing, hearing, and thinking things. If patients talk with words of sight, they will say things like, "I saw this as an opportunity." Then I use these same words to communicate back with them. "I see you want to make changes. How do you visualize change?" By using the patient's verbal patterns, I am able to create rapport. These are other examples of NLP in conversational forms:

I saw this as an opportunity to … (visual thinker)

I heard someone say … (auditory thinker)

That doesn't feel right. (emotional thinker)

I thought you said … (thoughtful thinker)

I felt like I was overheated. (emotional thinker)

Sounds good! (auditory thinker)

Being able to identify an individual's predominant thought processes helps us communicate with patients by being able to mirror back and match our communication using their predominant communication style. *I heard you say that you would like … I think you would like … You don't feel like … I heard you say …*

The Power of Words

Read the following words and pick the one that is most appealing: *constraint, limit, barrier, choice.*

Which word was it? Odds are it was 'choice' because the first three convey a feeling of negativity. Choice is associated with opportunity.

Words matter, so we need to choose them wisely. When thinking about how we relate to others, we need to be aware of the words we use. Are they negative or positive? Conscious awareness is required to process which words we put out into the conversation. They matter because they have an emotional attachment to them.

Similar words can feel differently. Think about the words baby and infant. While they have the same meaning, the word baby has more emotional power. If we say, "What a cute infant," it really doesn't have the same emotion as if we said, "What a cute baby." This is NLP, studying the effects of the words we use and learning how to create words to gain others' rapport.

I like to use expressive words like excited, happy, beautiful, respect, healing, and love. These are my words. I use them over and over again; they are habitual now.

Breaking Rapport

Other types of personalities to consider are the patients who are overly expressive, going on and on, over and over the same thing. With these patients, we need to actually *break rapport*. If I find myself in a position where someone needs to be interrupted, I start by doing the opposite of everything I see them doing. I go in reverse. If their arms are folded, I fold and unfold my arms. If they are high-pitched talkers, I begin to lower my voice and talk more slowly, which makes them stop and listen. If they are using direct eye contact, I let my eyes gaze around, then direct contact, then gaze. This is called *breaking rapport* with them. Doing this provides a slight mental shock to the other person, causing them to slow down and listen.

NLP: Helping Health Professionals Cope with Stress

Stress and burnout are serious concerns for the welfare of our health care workers. We need to stay in touch with how we are doing when providing care for ourselves and others. Are you experiencing any burnout? Is burnout in your near future?

A study done in 2017 by Kronos Incorporated[3] polled 257 registered nurses working in U.S. hospitals. The following statistics were revealed:

- 98% of hospital nurses reported their work was physically and emotionally demanding.
- 85% of the surveyed group said their work made them fatigued overall.
- 63% of the nurses noted that their work has resulted in nurse burnout.

- 44% reported being worried that their tiredness will cause their patient care to suffer.

- 41% of the surveyed group have considered changing hospitals in the past year (2017) due to burnout.

In a recent nationwide survey, almost half of the nurses surveyed indicated they were thinking of leaving their profession. A physician study quoted that 73% of physicians felt burnout enough to make them want to quit practicing medicine. When physicians were asked if they had ever felt burnout in their careers, 92% said yes.

Reducing Burnout Possibilities

Can incorporating NLP techniques into our job performance reduce the likelihood of burnout?

A study was done in 2016 on the effect of neuro-linguistic programming on occupational stress in critical care nurses (Masumeh HemmatiMaslakpak, Masumeh Farhadi, and Javid Fereidoni). The average baseline score of job stress was 120.88 and 121.36 for both the intervention and control groups. The control group received no NLP training. The experimental group was instructed on NLP techniques. The group that received NLP training reduced their stress scores to 64.53, while that of the control group remained relatively unchanged (120.96). The results showed that the use of NLP can increase coping with stressful situations, and it can reduce the adverse effects of occupational stress.

NLP allows us to connect with our patients by building a connection—both physical and emotional. When we add NLP to our toolbox, we remove barriers to care and allow compassion to shine through. These techniques can help us speak to patients so that they can hear, listen, and process.

How we see and feel toward others is the biggest connecting factor in nurse-to-patient relationships. It creates an atmosphere of hope and understanding. It saves time when we get in alignment with patients' needs by honoring effective communications. Each encounter with a patient has clues and messages. Learning to observe the messages and use them to create a space for mutual respect and acceptance is where the fun begins.

The Eyes Have It

Let the eyes be a clue as well. For example, you are helping a patient learn about diabetes. You ask them questions after you have explained what it is. You notice they look up and to the right. When patients look up and to the right, they are visual thinkers. By applying NLP, you are able to determine they are visual learners and that you need to write or draw the information in pictures so they can 'see' the diagrams. When they look side to side, they are audible learners, and you need to have them repeat the directions back to you. If they look down, they are kinesthetic, and you need to engage them in an activity so they can feel it; maybe you have them do the blood sugar testing with you.

It Takes All Kinds

Some of our patients only get the big picture. If you give them too much detail, they feel overloaded. I have to be very careful with this because overload can be my dominant way of communicating. If I'm being observant and using NLP, I can almost see the patient turn the knob to off and stop listening. Even for people who want to get the big picture, too much information in too little time is overwhelming.

In contrast, someone who wants to know the nitty-gritty details will get frustrated if you only present them with the big picture. When that detailed patient comes in, I have to get the paper out and write it all down. I must change my approach because they cannot interpret big picture ideas.

When styles are different, it can be challenging. I have a patient who comes in with a chart of all of his blood pressure and lab work results from over the years. He categorizes them so he can compare them each visit. He wants detailed explanations of each item—my head goes whoosh. I have to focus to stay with him because this goes against my natural tendency to think big. I have to take a deep breath and slow down so I can explain things in detail. It's important to him. It feels so tedious to me. It takes all kinds.

The Gift of NLP

Today, NLP offers scripts to help patients make changes. In *Consulting with NLP*, author Lewis Walker offers a complete process to incorporate NLP into your practice. When I first started with NLP, I wrote the scripts on index cards and kept them inside my folding medication pad. I would get them out and read them, sometimes right in front of the patients. They never seemed to notice. I encourage you to use this great educational tool.

Does it Work?

A while back, a 40-year-old patient came into the office who hadn't been in for two years. During those two years, she had quit smoking, left her husband, lost weight and looked great. She told me the last time she saw me in the office, she had been on Family Medical Leave (FMLA) and didn't want to go back to work because of stress and anxiety. She told me that I emphasized how important it was for her to get rid of the stress in her life. I said work was never going to change and if the job was stressing her out, then she needed to decide if that was the place for her. She said I suggested she try NLP to help her see things in her life differently. (I have no recollection of that visit.) She went crazy looking up information on NLP, and she began to make changes in her life. She quit her stressful job and got rid of a husband who was bringing her down. She quit smoking, started working out, met a wonderful new man and is happier than she has ever been! She said, "You shared NLP, and I took it to another level. I applied it to my life, and it changed everything. I love NLP." True story.

I was thrilled that she had studied it and applied it to her life. Her words to me were, "I am so grateful for you. NLP changed my life." She changed her life and mine. I believe that we are here to plant seeds using the tools we learn like NLP. Each time a client comes in, we reseed until wellness begins to bud. It is beautiful seeing flowers blossom. I want to shout out, "Keep supplying the seeds! Patients eventually will get it."

Practice Until it is Second Nature

Once we decide to focus on what we hear, feel, see, think, and how we behave, we begin to embed the process of being a better version of ourselves and helping others become a better version of themselves. We are all connected in how we see, hear, feel, and think about the world. I believe we can impart more positivity, more belief in healing, more feelings of well-being. To do this, to make this our dominant response, we must practice until it becomes second nature. If we try NLP for one day and think that it will be a part of who we are, we will be gravely mistaken. We must practice, think about it, feel the emotions of the conversations, and question everything. For example, when I feel anxious, I ask, "What is this about? What is upsetting me? Whose energy is it?" Then I listen to my answers. The listening is equally important!

Learn to Read People

Observe. Next time you go into a room or meet a new person, ask: Who are they being? How are they communicating verbally and nonverbally?

Pay attention. Ask, "How do I feel being around this person? How can I connect and engage them in a loving and healthy discussion with a positive outcome?"

Use mirroring and matching. Use their body dynamics, voice reflections, and their inner dialogue techniques. Follow their eye movement. Find out if they are emotional, visual, auditory, or a thinker. Then lead them into hopeful loving conversation.

Learn to use what you see, hear, feel, and think.

Learn About Yourself

Answering the following questions will be interesting and useful as you get more familiar with how you and others communicate.

- Assess your own communication style. Do you use words like think, see, hear, feel? What is your preferred way to communicate, e.g., verbal, in writing, one-on-one?

- Watch your family and identify their communication styles.

- Apply mirroring and matching to interactions with other people, e.g., at the dinner table and at work, and note what happens.

- Listen for clues from your patients to decide how they will receive communication from you. Clues will help you determine if they are visual, auditory, kinesthetic, or thought-provoked communicators.

- Use the techniques in reverse to break barriers that are negative.

Chapter Five

The Thinking-Linking Brain

There is nothing either good or bad but thinking makes it so.
—Shakespeare

The world as we have created it is a process of our thinking. It cannot be changed without changing our thinking.
—Albert Einstein

My Childhood

When I was 12 years old, I moved into a new house in a new neighborhood. I started a new school that was filled with people I didn't know. It wasn't long until I discovered that there were several girls there that did not like me who went on to boldly bully me. I often felt my stomach churning before I would go to school. A sense of dread filled me. Sometimes in the middle of school, I would get so sick to my stomach that I would start throwing up and get sent home. This was the beginning of me not feeling 'good enough.'

Then, shortly after our move, the next bombshell came. My mother met a man at work and within a few months, they were engaged to be married. My world felt scary all over. School was scary, my new stepdad, Don, was scary, and our new neighborhood was scary. My sister moved out when Don moved in, and he brought his daughter with him. It was a time of great changes. I was a very emotional kid, and all of this change embedded a lot of fear and feelings of uncertainty.

My mom and Don argued all of the time, and this became one of my greatest challenges in life. The years that followed were filled with the two of them bickering; it's how they got along for 40 years. They both loved me, but the stress caused me to lock myself in my room at night to get away from them.

When I got into nursing school, the loneliness and fear began to resurface. School was hard, and the harder it got, the more negative my feelings and thinking became. Eventually, I was not eating and lost 15 pounds. It was the only thing that I had control over. I knew that my behavior was destructive, but it was my mindset at the time.

Once I began taking psychology classes, I realized that my mindset was a mess. Slowly, I tried to incorporate what I was learning to become healthier and happier. It helped that I had a rotation at the hospital with patients who had severe depression. I remember a patient who was 15 years old. He never spoke a word to anyone. He came from a very affluent family in St. Louis. I always thought money could buy you anything, but he proved me wrong. I would just sit with him and talk to him. But I saw that he was blank. Nothing registered in his eyes. I think through meeting him, I was reminded of how alive I was and that if I wanted to get better, I needed to do the work. It tripped my switch, and I began to work on myself using the very techniques that I learned to help other people. I could not reach him and thought this was so strange at the time, but now I know that psychiatric disorders have many different levels.

Nursing school saved me. I decided I had to begin to challenge my own thoughts, which meant I had to become more conscious and aware so I could monitor my inner dialogue, catch it, trap it, repel it, and reverse it into love and positivity. This was never accomplished fully; the brain is a tricky thing.

Nursing provided me with a matrix for thinking differently. I saw people differently. I met people, and I truly wanted to know and help them. I think now it was because I wanted to truly know and help myself. Nursing taught me the crux of being human is to love and to serve. My education taught me that we create our realities, and if anyone gets better, it's because they try.

Helping Ourselves and Others Heal

How do we help ourselves and others heal? My journey through the 'stinking thinking' started in nursing school and is ongoing today. In the beginning, I dabbled here and there, but for the last 10 years, I have been very serious. I spend my time trying to correct my negative thoughts. I want to see my world differently. I want to feel joy and happiness, and the only way to accomplish that is to thread the needle with positivity. The needle hole is little, and it takes patience to push the thread of love through.

Network of Neurons

The brain is a massive network of 100 billion cells that communicate to billions of their colleagues, creating a network of a quadrillion connections that guide everything we do—all within this itty-bitty, 3-pound organ. It's amazing how much recall it has regarding memories, feelings, emotions, and visualizations.

Furthermore, if what we think and feel is in our unconscious, aka emotional brain, that means much of our behaviors are child-like, driven by action-orientated emotions we learned a long time ago.

The brain houses 90 billion neurons. Controlling it is not necessary because it works all on its own. We live 10% of our day in the conscious mind, awake and present in our lives. We live 90% of our day in the unconscious mind, replaying old memories and reels. This means we speak before we think, we feel before we express emotions. We spin in a cycle of recurrences, unless we start rethinking *thinking.*

Memory Cells

Our brain stores trauma and pain in memory cells. These memories only come up when we are pressured, scared, or fearful. These memories are our coping strategies, the learned behavior from the past that tell us what to think and feel when stress arises. The sounds of fear, rejection, and loneliness are recorded in our brains, and when the sympathetic fight-or-flight response is triggered, we go to the stored sounds and replay the lyrics. We get stuck in old memories and old emotions. We continue to wire and fire the same neurons over and over again, which only reinforces the memories and emotions.

This is important because when we are stressed out, our stress response is activated. Whether after a car accident that is causing severe back pain or in the hospital coping with unexpected illness, patients bring along their imperfect past and learned fear behaviors.

Guess who gets to soothe them, put the fire out? Wonderful nurses. We are there with the patients, we care for them, talk to them, listen to them, soothe them. The nastiest patients are usually the ones who have the most painful past. Why? Because they are triggered by their fear, and they want to protect themselves.

Brain Functions

Dr. Joe Dispenza tells us that "What is wired together fires together. We are what we think." Think about this. If we live in constant negativity, we generate more negative neurons. If we live with positivity, we generate more positive neurons. Unfortunately, science confirms that we are negative a great deal of our day. The National Science Foundation reports that an average person has about 12,000 to 60,000 thoughts per day. Of those, 80% are negative and 95% are repetitive thoughts, the same thoughts today as we had yesterday, and the day before that.

I first learned about thinking and linking in the brain at one of Joyce Meyer's conferences. Her guest speaker was Dr. Caroline Leaf who discussed how thinking wires and fires in our brains. She presented a picture of a beautiful tree that was green and healthy and another tree with no buds, no leaves—just dried out branches. She described that every time we have a negative thought, we reinforce those thoughts in our brain, creating and reinforcing the dried-up branches. The brain wiring therefore learns negativity, learns sadness, learns fear. To change our brains, we have to do something different. We have to think differently, catch ourselves in negativity and redirect it to positivity. This means we have to learn, read, study, and listen to things that can increase the amount of time we spend creating a different future response. We have to create a life that supports us by learning and creating positive emotions—the beautiful blooming tree.

Energy is Everything

I remember working as a floater at the hospital after graduating from nursing school. One of the most disturbing experiences I had was being assigned to the psychiatric floor. My duties were to assist the patients throughout the Electroconvulsive Therapy (ECT) procedures. While I learned about it in nursing school, I had never seen anything like it. My first time, I went to the patient's room and another nurse helped me move a gentleman onto the gurney. He was blank, without expression, and already slightly tranquilized. I wheeled him to the treatment room. They began to apply large electrode wires to his temples in preparation for shock therapy. Once they inserted a mouth guard, they cleared the table of all employees. The doctor then pressed a red switch that applied electrical voltage to the patient's brain. Following the jolt, the patient went into a massive convulsion, flopping all over the table, followed by a death-like stillness. My heart was racing as I just stood there in shock and disbelief.

After the procedure, it was my job to monitor the patient until he woke up. When he awakened, I put him in a wheelchair and took him to the cafeteria to eat. At the cafeteria tables sat other patients who also had received ECT treatments that morning. They all looked like zombies methodically eating their breakfast. Flat, unemotional, sitting silently while they ate. It was heartbreaking.

I was 24 years old when I witnessed such depression that electric shocks had to be applied to release the negative thinking, the suicidal ideation, and the angry behaviors that medication could not control.

I got pulled there often and saw repeat patients. I felt so much empathy for these patients. What could make them so sad? My consolation was to hold their hand and speak softly and sweetly. Even as I write this now, the image seems so inhuman.

When I became a nurse practitioner, I learned that when people come in with depression, there is always another underlying issue. It is very rare that I see someone with depression who doesn't have a story of abuse, neglect, harassment, abandonment or some type of history of post-traumatic stress syndrome. I can empathize with them because I have seen the depth of depression firsthand. My life before I was 20 was streaked with fear, abandonment, rejection, and hate. These became valuable lessons for who I am, who I want to be, and how I can help others going through the same things.

Stored Stress

Stresses create memories that are stored in our brains. Whenever we connect with a stressful situation, our brain goes, "Where have I seen this before? Oh, that's right, run for your life!" Then the brain goes into panic mode. All of the old memories come flooding back with feelings—without our permission.

The hospital setting is notorious for creating stress. Patients' blood sugars go up, their blood pressure goes up, and the risk of infection and blood clots go up. When patients get into the hospital, they lose their independence, and it creates a knee-jerk reaction.

Their stress behaviors become apparent when they start to become demanding, put the call light on constantly, seem bothered by you walking in, are unsure if they want to take their medications, or just won't get out of bed to walk or sit in their chair.

All of the makings for fear are present in the hospital. As providers, we have to remind ourselves that patients come with a whole load of past experiences and a built-in fight-or-flight response. Once they get put in the hospital, they cannot control their fight/flight reactions. They are stuck in the bed and cannot run away. They want things they cannot have, and their stress response is in overdrive.

I think hospitals should have a therapy staff, and every patient gets assigned a therapist, someone they can talk to throughout their visit at the hospital. Sometimes we use clergy for this, but a trained hospital therapist would be awesome.

In the meantime, nurses have to be there to calm and quiet the patients.

Perceptions

Perception is the state of being or process of becoming aware of something through the senses. What we feel, hear, smell, touch, and taste all convert into neurons processed by our brains. They convert into thoughts that drive our choices and actions.

It is interesting that "two people can have the exact same external experience with profoundly different internal reactions, based on the structure and patterning of their nervous system." (Leavek) Again, this means our reactions are learned behaviors, and in order to be different, we have to begin to think differently.

Worrying—Such a Waste

Other interesting brain work discovered by scientists is that 85% of what we worry about never happens. With the 15% of the worries that did happen, 79% of the subjects discovered that either they could handle the difficulty better than expected, or that the difficulty taught them a lesson worth learning. The conclusion is that 97% of our worries are baseless and result from an unfounded pessimistic perception (that repetitive thinking problem). (Leahy, 2005, Study of Cornell University).

Knowing these statistics, what if part of our normal care plan was to give our patients a few relaxation tips that help them focus on their thought processes and create positive energy? I know, it's a huge 'what if,' but one worth considering.

As Albert Einstein stated so eloquently: *Everything is energy and that's all there is to it. Match the frequency of the reality you want, and you cannot help but get that reality. It can be no other way. This is not philosophy. This is physics.*

Thus, thinking makes it so.

Karma or The Law of Cause and Effect

Randall E. Burton wrote, "Today's seed. Tomorrow's harvest."

The idea that we reap what we sow has much to do with the type of energy we send out into the universe, where and how it gathers momentum, and how it returns to us as either positive or negative energy.

When I am being negative, I tell myself that every thought is like a prayer, and ask myself, "Is this what I want to pray for?" I have been known to say that to patients as well. The response is always "no." I then encourage myself and my patients to plant new seeds of hope.

I have learned that 'hurting people hurt people.' I use this quote to manage our medical office. When patients come in and yell about their copay, I remind the receptionist that it is not about them. The patient is hurting, maybe physically, emotionally, or financially, and they are expressing it outwardly through their negative behaviors. I tell staff, "Do not accept negative energy; it is not about you."

When I began to learn to see others' pain, I realized that their pain and yelling triggered my past emotional pains. Suddenly I am being yelled at by my stepdad and I want to defend myself. When I learned that their yelling is about them and not me, I was able to listen and become empathetic as well as settle down my stress response.

Each of us has to uncover what part of ourselves is being triggered by others' behavior, and then self-correct, so that we don't hold onto the negative energy.

Masaru Emoto Water Crystals

I love the work of Masaru Emoto.[4] He concentrates on water crystal formation by using prayer, both positive and negative. He prays over the water molecules, then he looks at them under the microscope to analyze the type of crystals that form. After repetitive work in this field, he is able to document that positive thinking creates beautiful crystals and negative thinking creates ugly crystals. Before we scoff, consider that up to 90% of our blood is water and 60% of our body is water. What kind of crystals are we making through thought alone?

New Tricks Toolbox

There are a number of additional tools that prove old dogs can learn new tricks. Become aware of what you are negative about. Question it and where it came from in your past. Then turn it around and ask yourself what you learned from that experience and how it made you a better person.

Byron Katie:

Look up her work online to get her workbook. I have had amazing thought patterns reversed using *The Work of Byron Katie*[5] to question negative thoughts.

1. Is it true? (Yes or no. If no, move to question c.)
2. Can you absolutely know that it's true? (Yes or no.)
3. How do you react and what happens when you believe that thought?
4. Who or what would you be without the thought?

Wayne Dyer:

- How others treat me is their path, how I react is mine.

- Change the way you look at things, and the things you look at change.

- What is the difference between good and God? A zero or an "o." So whatever makes you feel good inside, that is God.

Dr. Joe Dispenza:

- Reduce stress because it wipes out your ability to move forward.

- Close your eyes and see yourself in the future magically going through life in love and acceptance.

- Acknowledge that if your thoughts can make you sick (stress and emotional), then your thoughts also can make you well.

- Get rid of your emotional addiction to negativity. You don't need it anymore.

The Silva Method: [6] Learn mind control. Start by closing your eyes and mentally place a movie screen in front of you. Place the problem in the middle of the screen. Then begin to create the solution to the left of the main screen problem. Focus on the new image of the solution. Then, to the left of the last image, imagine the solution as complete.

Learn about hypnosis and make an audio of yourself creating the life you want. I like to listen to my audio before I go to bed when I am entering the alpha and theta brain waves.

Start your day with positivity. Open your eyes and say thank you. Listen to motivational videos shortly after opening your eyes. My favorites are Tony Robbins, Les Brown, and Dr. Joe Dispenza.

Create a song library that is upbeat and motivational. Listen to it every day. Music is joy.

Read over the Oath of Manifestation. I recorded it on my phone and listen to it in my meditation practices or when I work out.

Make your own incantation card and record it. Listen to it twice a day.

Use Mind Mapping[7] techniques to map out your solutions, ideas, or plans on how to change your future or negative thinking.

Practice, practice, practice! Do you remember how you learned your multiplication tables or rehearsed your ABCs? Through rehearsal and repetition. If you want to do something different, you have to rehearse it until it becomes automatic. Or, as Vincent Lombardi said, "Practice makes permanent."

The Thinking-Linking Brain

I'm going to conclude this chapter by circling back to the concept that *what we wire together, fires together.* The success of any change management tool, process or behavioral technique depends first and foremost on our conscious desire to change, then secondly on our ability to define what is not working, and why.

We have to metaphorically untangle the cords and knots so we can rewire ourselves, so we have an uncontaminated, clear connection to our energy, and the energy of the universe. We have to script positive rehearsals, then practice, practice, practice to embed new patterns and habits. It takes time for them to become our natural, preferred patterns and behaviors.

What new tricks are you adding to your toolbox?

Chapter Six

The One You Feed

Be a student to those above you, be a teacher to those below you,
be a fellow traveler to those at your side.
–Unknown

We are the sum total of our experiences, which is to say that we
are burdened by our pasts. When we experience stress or fear in
our lives, if we would look carefully, we would find that the cause is
actually a memory. It is the emotions which are tied to these mem-
ories which affect us now. The subconscious associates an action
or person in the present with something that happened in the past.
When this occurs, emotions are activated, and stress is produced.
–Morrnah Nalamaku Simeona

Our Physical Response to an Emotional Experience

Working in the Emergency Room (ER) provided me with a lot of life
experiences and emotional growths. I was a young mom back then,
and at the same time, I was learning how to handle ER traumas.
Our ER had radios that we used to communicate with the paramedics in the field. When we had patients coming in an ambulance, the
paramedics would call us on our emergency radio system to alert us
about the condition of the patient they were bringing in. This system
allowed us to get the trauma room ready with the necessary equip-
ment and staff that the patients would need on arrival.

I clearly remember one disturbing afternoon. The paramedics
called in; the radio started chirping and vibrating throughout the whole

emergency room. The doctor put the system on speaker and the words rang out, "We have a 12-year-old male found unconscious on the playground laboring for air … " With that I was off to the races, and my adrenaline began to pump. Off I went to get the trauma room ready. I waited nervously with the doctor and nurses when a scrawny 12-year-old boy was rapidly wheeled in. He was not responding to verbal or physical stimulation. We began the work up. He had a normal head CT scan. His head and neck X-rays also were normal. No foreign body was in his airway. His lab work all came back normal, too.

I was perplexed by what was the matter with this little guy when all of his tests kept coming back normal. I watched the pediatrician, awaiting his next orders, as he looked at the little guy in deep concentration. Suddenly, he told us to give him Ativan IV push. I was surprised by this order, but I was quick to get the medication started. I thought to myself, "How is this going to help?"

Sure enough, within minutes of receiving the Ativan, the little guy began to perk up. What in the world was going on here? I was confused! Later, I learned that the doctor had diagnosed the boy with a panic attack, which resulted in a loss of consciousness. I also found out that the boy was being bullied on the playground, and he became so alarmed that he suffered a severe panic attack. The mom in me was heartbroken for that boy. I just couldn't believe it. Physical symptoms from emotional pain, one of the paradoxical traps of stress and emotions.

The Stress Trap

Writing about stress comes naturally to me. I feel like I have spent so much of my life in its grasp. Because of the different stresses I experienced in my youth, I easily can allow myself to get bombarded by stress in my day-to-day activities. The older I get, the more purposeful I have to be to resist the temptation to fall into the stress trap.

I am not alone. Over 72% of physicians and 35.5% of nurses currently are experiencing emotional exhaustion. Nurses are more inclined to have intense depersonalization at 54.2%. Nurses also have a double incidence of depression as compared to the national average in the United States.

This part of the book focuses on helping us learn that we are normal, stress is normal, and that it is mandatory to have a plan of action when it comes. Stress is always lurking, ready to come crashing down on us. We need to get prepared by learning calming approaches and by staying persistent in our practices. As we learn to build our resistance to stress, we can then plant the seeds for our families, friends, and patients to de-stress too.

Years ago, I hit the Mack truck of stress. It changed me forever. I had to look at how I wanted to live my life and who was going to be in control of it. Me or the other guy.

At that time, I owned a family medical practice, and it was my mission to make everybody happy. In reality, that can never happen, but I believed I could. No matter how many meetings and staff pow wows I held, I could not get the staff to love each other. We had two employees fuming at each other every day.

Eventually the situation became unbearable. The tension in the office was so stifling. I was at the point where I didn't want to go to work anymore—and I owned the practice! One evening after everyone else had left, I was confronted with a hysterical and angry woman who very emotionally shouted out, "I cannot work with her anymore! I am going to hurt her!"

I realized at that moment the severity of what was going on. I had to admit that she was having more angry days than not, and while she worked hard and was smart, something had to change before something bad happened. I had to let her go. When I fired her, I was stunned by how it made me feel inside, like I had just been through shock treatment. I was shaking inside and numb on the outside.

Weeks later I got a letter in the mail that she had made charges against me. I cried when I read the letter and all of the things that I was accused of in it. I was deeply hurt. I would go home after work, go to bed, get up, eat dinner, then go back to bed and sleep until the next morning. This went on for several weeks. What in the world was wrong with me? I literally shut down emotionally; I could not force myself to function in the evenings.

Over the next few years, I experienced a lot. A billing company didn't bill our services and lost us thousands of dollars, two of my collaborative physicians died suddenly, and the paperwork began to quadruple after the new health care bills passed. I started to feel panic, have racing thoughts, and wonder about my sanity.

I'd seen how devastating depression and anxiety were on my patients, and I was experiencing it firsthand. I now could understand why so many people wanted to sedate their pain with Xanax.

Root Causes

Emotional traumas, stress response, depression, anxiety, and panic attacks are the root cause of approximately 60% to 80% of all office visits and hospitalizations. Some sources say it is even as high as 90%.

According to a 2012 article in *JAMA Internal Medicine*, "44% of Americans reported an increase in psychological stress over the past five years." Just imagine where that must be in today's climate.

Interestingly, even though stress levels are up and visits to the office and hospital are highly stress-related, those of us in the medical field rarely address it with our patients. In a study done by the National Center for Biotechnology Information from 2006-2009, only 3% of 33,045 office visits included stress management counseling by the patients' primary care physicians. Stress management counseling was the least common type of all counseling. What a shame.

Evidence exists that obesity, diabetes, hypertension, and many other diseases can be deeply rooted in stress-related, psychological imbalances. Yet, if providers only discuss stress issues with patients 3% of the time, then we clearly are not addressing the root cause of illnesses in which stress is an underlying issue as much as 90% of the time.

We are medicating the psychological problems with weight, diabetes, and hypertension drugs but, unfortunately, not with stress management techniques and counseling. Antidepressants and antianxiolytics account for 10 of the top 50 drugs on the market, and that doesn't count how many antacids, antihypertensives or sleeping pills that are prescribed for what really equates to mood disorders. As nurses and providers, we need to become empowered to address these issues. We can! We can begin to make an impact on an issue that is penetrating every aspect of our health care system today: STRESS!

The first step: heal thyself by learning about how stress and burnout play into our own lives. Next, help others. *Learn one technique, teach one, master one.* Be the hope you need, and the hope others need.

Chronic Stress Response

What does the body do with stress and emotions? It creates hormones in an attempt to provide homeostasis. On the outside it may look like we are coping with stress, but there is no homeostasis going on inside of our cells. The cells are saturated with over 1,400 stress chemicals, all of which cause an up regulation of our bodies' fight, flight or freeze response. Worry and stress can show up in patients' labs, too. I often see elevated levels of glucose, ferritin, uric acid, C-Reactive Protein (CRP), and homocysteine. We can see it in their vital signs, hear the stress in their voices, and over time, observe their vulnerability to infections, headaches, and insomnia. The list goes on and on.

When the body feels, sees, hears or even recalls stress, it automatically can cascade into our built-in stress response. The first responder is the amygdala, which is located in the brain. Its function is similar to a switchboard operator. It defines the incoming emotion and if it is an emergency, it stimulates the hypothalamus, located in the brain as well. The hypothalamus reacts by activating the pituitary gland, which produces hormones that stimulate the adrenal glands, which produce cortisol and epinephrine. The stress slides around the vagus nerve connecting electrical circuits so they are ready to fire "run for your life."

Now, imagine this is going on day and night. One stress response jumping to the next. The body is set to a timer of negative emotions. Our precious nervous system is being damaged, becoming fragile from hormonal and chemical overstimulation. This leads to numerous life-threatening diseases. Almost any disease can be triggered by chronic elevations of stress hormones and maladaptation of coping strategies.

The immune system also gets involved with the stress response so it can protect us. The immune system calls in the artillery, but eventually it gets exhausted and inflammation sets in.

We may see this as coughs and colds, asthma attacks, rheumatoid flares, fibromyalgia, or autoimmune diseases and inflammation. The body can't keep up with all of the incoming stress intruders. It gets tired. Then we develop dysfunction or disease. Sex is out, our energy level is low, the weight creeps up. Sometimes we can't sleep and sometimes all we want to do is sleep. Arteries are getting thick and stiff. Our body cannot detox. Our bowels slow down or speed up. Our blood sugars go all over the place. We go from wired to tired and then can't figure out why we feel bad all of the time.

A healthy body relies on the nervous system, endocrine system, and immune system to be in balance. When stress hits, the whole system goes haywire. With the mere thought of a stressful situation, the body can go on autopilot to create the necessary stress hormones that are supposed to help us find balance, but balance isn't a thing anymore. The body is worn out. Disease sets in. The end. Or is it? Can we do something about it?

Learned Stress Response

Marilyn came in for one of her frequent-flyer appointments for stress and anxiety. She was a beautiful young woman, smart, had a great job and was raising three small children with no child support. Whenever she comes in, she makes me laugh. She is boisterous and all out there. I love her. Initially, she was coming in for headaches. Then she started having stomach issues. Each time, I kept telling her it was stress. She refused to listen to my assessment; she was "fine."

As her symptoms continued, she confided in me that she would get to work and sit in the parking lot and cry, then call in sick and go home. On and off for a year, she struggled with this. I tried to give her medications, I tried getting her into therapy, but she just didn't feel she needed it. Her direct comment to me was, "It's my job!"

Eventually she quit her job thinking that all of her problems would suddenly go away.

Months later, she resurfaced again feeling stress and crying in the parking lot at her new job. We had a long discussion about her emotional care. It wasn't that she hated her job as much as she was stressed in her personal life. Her childhood consisted of being homeless, living in a car with her mother and siblings. She thought the job was making her crazy, but the crazy was already embedded in her from early on. She learned her mother's stressful coping strategies. Her dysregulated stress response was created at a very early age. The job definitely was pushing her learned stress buttons that caused her to feel crazy. But in the end, she had to come to terms with the stress and anxiety that was inside of her that she had never attempted to control before. Part of the issue was that her stress was a learned behavior, but it was also a behavior and feeling that she had most of her life. On the outside looking in, she was fun, interesting, lively, and awesome to work with, but inside her, the fear of abandonment was killing her. After two years of feeling crazy and going through two jobs, she finally was willing to see a psychiatrist and get the help she needed.

Stress could be considered a memory that lies dormant until we have our next stressful event. Then the memory of the old stress is triggered, and the old adaptation skills resurface, creating physical, mental, and emotional havoc. We are not commonly taught how to deal with stress correctly. The body just doesn't know what to do, so it resorts to creating stress hormones to help balance out the body.

Please consider the stress response next time you are faced with an uptight patient or family member. Ask yourself, "I wonder what underlying stress response is at work here?"

Our Inability to Adapt

Regrettably with stress, the incoming negative stimuli generally trump the positive. Furthermore, stress can show up even when there isn't really an emergency. We may just think there is or worry one into existence. It doesn't matter to the brain if it is real or imagined, the response is the same: "Run for your life, quick."

People feel fear about perceived or remembered events. A boy who was bitten by a dog freaks out whenever he sees a dog. It doesn't matter that the dog is not biting him, the memory holds onto the stress.

Martin Seligman, founder of positive psychology, researched learned helplessness. In his studies with dogs, he was able to induce helplessness by repeating negative stimuli that the dogs were unable to get away from. Eventually the dogs gave up trying to avoid the stimuli and just let it happen. When the dogs were moved to a new situation where they could easily escape the negative stimuli, they didn't even try.

Seligman's theory is that when people think they can't do something to change a bad situation, they give up and stop trying. How is that okay?

Some patients who come in with depression are in a state of learned helplessness, and no matter what we do, they are just not willing to try to get better. They just can't.

When we encounter a noncompliant patient and ask ourselves, "What is the underlying issue?" we may need to step up and ask some difficult questions. As health care providers, something we say can make a difference, sooner or later. We become the stimulus, the seed so to speak. If we continue to fertilize their health each visit, eventually they may get excited to create a new health goal.

To me, Martin Seligman's ideas prove that we are more of a magnet for the negative things in life than the positive. It's why the stories on the news have such an impact. Our brains are programmed for survival, so when we hear or read a story that we perceive could threaten our survival, we tell it to other people. By repeating the story, we perpetuate our anxiety and negativity, wiring and firing that stress response within ourselves. Then the stress response becomes strengthened. This just breeds more helplessness and hopelessness. It becomes a vicious cycle.

Stopping the Cycle

The Story of Two Wolves[8]

An old Cherokee is teaching his grandson about life. "A fight is going on inside me," he said to the boy. "It is a terrible fight, and it is between two wolves. One is evil—he is anger, envy, sorrow, regret, greed, arrogance, self-pity, guilt, resentment, inferiority, lies, false pride, superiority, and ego."

He continued, "The other is good—he is joy, peace, love, hope, serenity, humility, kindness, benevolence, empathy, generosity, truth, compassion, and faith. The same fight is going on inside you—and inside every other person, too."

The grandson thought about it for a minute and then asked his grandfather, "Which wolf will win?"

The old Cherokee simply replied, "The one you feed."

~

It's time to step back again. We've reviewed how our brains permanently store memories of negative responses, how we repeat learned behaviors when we experience stress, and how we submit to the stress chemicals flooding our bodies and brains. Now what? Giving up is not an option. If we learned helplessness, let's unlearn it. We have to practice doing and feeling things in a different way. We have to feed the *good wolf.*

If we continually talk about negative things, we become grounded in negatives. Just like being around a negative person can suddenly make us negative and defensive. We are absorbing their negative energy.

Hit the reverse button. Let's respond by redirecting our thoughts—and our patients'—simply by posing different questions.

For example, instead of answering the patient's question, "What if the operation doesn't work out?" propose a different question: "What if it does and you feel better than you have in a long time?"

If the question is "Why did I have a heart attack?" redirect it with, "Why did I survive a heart attack?" Maybe it is to go on to do greater things.

Where our focus goes, our mind flows. What if we asked patients this question: "What makes you feel grateful?" instead of asking "What is bothering you?"

Gratitude weeds out the negative. Gratitude gives the biggest contribution to happiness. There are approximately 420,000 study results on Google Scholar regarding the benefits of gratitude and happiness. What if we envisioned a new health care system that gave patients handbooks to help relieve stress while in the hospital or in everyday life? We give them uncountable other useless pieces of paper; why not give them something that promotes real healing? Page one would start with: "What makes you grateful?"

Which brings us back to "taking control of our emotion becomes our greatest mission." If we learn one technique to help ourselves, then when memories and learned beliefs show up, we can prevent old survival patterns from repeating over and over. What would happen if we asked ourselves and our patients, "Is there another way to look at this?" It's worth exploring.

Strategies of Winners

A few years ago, I went to Tony Robbins' seminar and learned his strategies to start the day as a winner. His strategies include three steps. The first is gratitude. For 3 minutes, you think of everything and anything you are grateful for. Then the next 3 minutes consist of prayer with a twist of positivity. This means you don't pray for healing, you pray, "Thank you for helping me feel great." Lastly, for 3 minutes you think about what you intend for your day or life. Dream big dreams, think loving thoughts, and plan the perfect day every day. I like to do this while I am meditating or running.

Vagus Nerve Strengthening

Use techniques that stimulate the vagus nerve to simmer the fire. Do head and neck exercises, toe touches and then bring your arms up over your head and breathe. All of these can realign your vagus responses. Straighten your spine with confidence. Try gargling for 15 seconds when you brush your teeth. Several times a day stimulate the vagus nerve in the back of the throat by humming, whistling, and singing. Who can be unhappy when they are singing and humming? How about whistling while you work? Add in a self-hug to connect with your feel-good oxytocin chemical.

Cortisol Awakening Response

Cortisol is not only related to stress, but also to normal functioning on a day-to-day basis. We can measure a cortisol awakening response (CAR). If someone is stressed, they may have a poor CAR, and there are some natural ways to balance your cortisol levels. Think cortisol issues when people complain of feeling tired when they wake up in the morning even after a full night of sleep.

There are ways to trigger a healthy cortisol response and improve our mood and fatigue levels. This can be done by jumping in place at the crack of dawn, jumping jacks, bouncing or dancing. After you complete a few minutes of movement, chug a full glass of water. Getting the body going first thing in the morning is essential to mood and mental salvation. Instruct patients to do these easy steps when they get up to realign their cortisol response. It's good, clean, and fun especially when your spouse or kids look at you like you're crazy.

Essential Oils

I love essential oils. I keep a bottle handy at work for people who need it. Sometimes those people are me or my staff. I will invite patients to try lavender oil if they seem stressed out in the office. I simply put a few drops in their hand and have them rub their hands together. Then I have them put their hands around their nose like a tent and just breathe in slowly, letting the essential oils penetrate. Relaxation occurs through the absorption of the oil by the olfactory nerve, which then stimulates the limbic system made up of our emotional centers in the amygdala and the hippocampus. Putting oil in a diffuser during the day is a nice way to work. If you want to use lavender to help you sleep, try applying it to the bottom of your feet at night. Our feet are home to the biggest pores of our bodies, so you get the best absorption. Many meridians or pathways of the body either begin or end in the feet. Chinese practitioners focus on the meridian centers in the feet, so go ahead and massage your feet.

Ask Better Questions

Utilize great questions that help provoke your brain to find a better solution. Author Noah St. John says if we ask better questions, our brain will look for better answers. Why do I have so many gifts to share with the world? Why am I the best group facilitator in the world? Why do I have a bestseller? Now think of some of your own. Consider what questions or visualization techniques your patients can use while you are doing painful procedures. Memorize one that you will always have handy.

Ruminations Prevention

In a study reviewing rumination, participants were asked to watch a very sad movie. Some were asked to ruminate on their own past pains and sadness, others to try to redirect their negative thoughts. Participants asked to ruminate with their thoughts kept their negative mood. The group of participants instructed to distract themselves showed a reduction in negative mood.

Tell your brain to shut up. Think of a time in your life that you were happy and successful. Concentrate on that. Have patients concentrate on the times they felt healthy and what that was like.

Food Styling

Choose foods that won't cause inflammation, i.e., reduce carbohydrates and gluten. Increase intake of vegetables, healthy fats, and fruits. Carbs are sugars that cause inflammation and increase our stress response.

Holy basil tea or green tea. Holy basil is a natural herb; studies show that it helps benefit a feeling of well-being.

Exercise is equal to taking one Prozac a day. It reduces inflammation, improves mood, and makes us feel stronger. Go Superwoman/man!

Learn one technique, teach one, master one.[9] Be the hope you need, then flip it and be the hope provider.

Chapter Seven

The Anatomy of Energy

If you want to find the secrets of the universe, think in terms of
energy, frequency and vibration.
—Nikola Tesla

I define connection as the energy that exists between people
when they feel they are seen, heard, and valued; when they can give
and receive without judgment; and when they derive sustenance and
strength from the relationship.
—Brené Brown

Our body is made up of energy that we cannot see. The energy is very similar to that of a cell phone. The call and the conversation happen without us ever seeing any sign of energy movement. But it is there: the cellular tower is directing the energy to our phones unbeknownst to us.

Just as the universe is filled with an energy matrix, we are energy-based beings. Energy makes our hearts beat, our lungs expand, and our blood circulate. There is also the energy of the thoughts we think, the love we create, and the flow of our spirit and soul.

When I see an individual who is sick, I ask, "Why are they losing energy?" Anemia and fibromyalgia are both diseases that can be quantified by the absence of energy. With these diseases, the body does not have enough electrical molecules to produce energy. Their fields are diminished.

If we start thinking in terms of energy issues, which can be functional, electrical, endocrine, hormonal, and immunological, then we will ask different questions. By exploring different options, we likely will get better answers to our questions.

We are all familiar with the electrical currents of the brain, heart, and lungs, but what about our energy centers? Energy is created in and around us. It is easy to see the energy of our breath but not easy to see the energy created by the foods we consume. We can sense our heart beating, but we cannot feel the propulsion of thought as energy. So how do we work with our energy systems to enhance our physical, emotional, and spiritual well-being?

We were born to be hunters and gatherers, to move and groove to the beat of survival. In the past, survival meant that we had to run, capture, kill, eat, sleep, and start all over again. Animals are smart: they stuck to the basics. They eat, drink, and exercise without overthinking or overworking. Humans added materialism, and now the hunting and gathering we do is for new cars and cell phones.

Yet, as humans, we function as mental, emotional, physical, and spiritual beings. We require balance in our lives, but most of the time, we are off balance, feel disconnected, and are fatigued because we are moving the brain and not the body. Until we begin to focus on our self-care, it will be difficult to live in joy, love, happiness, and health.

As both consumers and creators of our own body's energy, it's surprising how little attention so many of us pay to this vital resource. What do we do to consume and create energy? Let's start with the most obvious: exercise and nutrition.

Exercise and Nutrition

People do not always think of movement and exercise as an aspect of energy; however, exercising for even a brief period—enough to get the heart rate up and stretch, flex, move the body—improves mood, reduces inflammation, and makes us feel stronger. Our bodies were made to move, yet studies show that only about 23% of Americans meet the exercise recommendation in the United States.

Food is the energy source for our body. When we eat, food is turned into energy, creating adenosine triphosphate, or ATP, which is the fuel that makes our bodies run. When we lack sufficient exercise and have a poor diet, we succumb to pain, stiffness, depression, insomnia, and a variety of other ailments. Yet it remains challenging for us to build exercise and nutritious food into our routines because we don't think of them in the right terms. We need to think in terms of energy.

Emotional Benefits of Exercise

When I conduct seminars on weight and exercise, I love to speak to the emotional benefits of exercise. It has been hypothesized that exercise is the equivalent to taking Prozac, which contains the chemical that increases our serotonin in the brain to make us feel happy. There are numerous studies indicating that exercise has the ability to create new neurons in the brain and help support our moods, sleep cycles, energy, and outlook on life, as well as improve life longevity. The process of neurogenesis or creating new neurons through exercise is also a great form of keeping the brain healthy.

Exercise is recommended as a means to support the body and prevent the furthering disability of disease; unfortunately, it is not a first line prescription like medications. I automatically think to the patients with back pain or other sources of chronic pain; these patients end up doing less instead of what they need to do, which is stretch and move more, likely at a slower pace and non-aggressively. Chronic inactivity causes chronic immobility.

I personally can attest that exercise corrects mood and energy issues. It is part of my daily routine, and I cannot live without it. If I am on vacation, nothing happens until Donna has taken her morning run. This is because my brain needs exercise to feel good. I have tapped into the endorphins and dopamine surges through exercise and when I don't exercise, I lose these surges. I think everyone should jump on the running trail and make themselves some new neuropeptides. I love me some endogenous opioids for breakfast![10]

Like antidepressants, exercise also increases the synthesis of new neurons in the adult brain, a two- to three-fold increase in hippocampal neurogenesis.[11]

Lack of exercise is a chronic health condition. Maybe instead of the diagnosis diabetes, we should be calling it inactivitis. Of course, we don't have a drug for inactivitis. It is estimated that there are approximately 250,000 premature deaths per year in the United States that are considered to be highly correlated to physical inactivity. According to epidemiological data reviewed in "waging war on modern chronic diseases,"[12] physical inactivity increases the incidence of at least 17 unhealthy conditions, most of which are considered to be chronic diseases. When we see that longevity is going down instead of up, we need to back up and retrace our roots of health.

I learned about exercise firsthand. In college, I had a very small support system with minimal family interaction. Sometimes I felt alone and unfortunately, I had very few skills to balance life. I had a Bible, a pack of cigarettes, two good legs, and a brain to keep me going. I prayed a lot, marked in my Bible, and tried to think straight—which wasn't always easy.

I lived across the street from Forest Park in St. Louis, an amazingly beautiful park that easily allows connecting with the energy of outdoors. I would go there to study and to exercise. I started a running program to help ease the wackiness in my brain. When I was feeling stressed and captive in the dorm studying, I would head outdoors for a run to ease my anxiety. Sometimes I went to the dorm's gym in the basement to play loud music and dance to Michael Jackson's "Beat It." The gym became my dance floor, and I became connected to the music. I was surprised to learn that music stimulates both sides of our brain, and dancing pumps up energy centers. Dancing is great exercise, and it calms the vagus nerve.

Energy Guidance Network

As I got older, I began a new journey into energy—a kind of energy I had never heard of before: the energy of auras, chakras, and meridians. I was never taught this in school or other social circles, so initially, I just wrote it off as unscientific. But it kept coming at me, and I became very curious. I was struggling spiritually and feeling emotionally drained from my work, which is a bad but all too common combination in the field of medicine. After I got my first dose of energy work, I began to crave more.

I made an appointment to do energy work with a lovely friend of my sister-in-law named Julie. She practices Pranic Healing. When I walked into the room for my first session, I was unsure of what to expect. Then I saw a picture of Jesus hanging on the wall and was relieved that this wasn't going to be some antichrist technique. Julie's smile was infectious, and her voice was happy and soothing. I felt at ease right away.

I laid down on the warmed table, and Julie explained how energy work helps us heal. She turned the lights down, soft music played in the background, and all of the parts of my body relaxed. Julie, using her Pranic techniques, cleaned my auras and energy centers and prayed over me. For an hour, I was in a deep meditative state. When I was done, I felt amazing. I signed up for another session. After my second session with Julie, I wanted to learn how to do this work for myself and my patients. Luckily, Julie wasn't only a practitioner, but also a teacher of Pranic Healing. I signed up and took her class.

I asked my niece to let me practice my newly learned energy work on her. She was open to it, and I was so grateful. With love and patience, I began my work of cleaning her energy and restoring her beautiful aura. She was relaxed and breathed easily. When we were finished, I asked her what she thought. She loved it. She told me, "I love that thing you did over my body. It just made me feel so calm." People don't understand that their bodies are full of energy that might be blocked. Energy work involves multiple layers.[13]

Energy Centers[14]

The energy of our aura, our chakra systems, and our meridian systems is part of our energy guidance network. Restoring balance to these systems helps us maintain and restore health.

Auric Field: The aura is an electromagnetic field that surrounds our body. Aura in Greek means 'breeze.' Auras flow around anything that has an energetic vibration, like humans, animals, and plants. The auric field has seven layers that all connect to one of our seven chakras. These energy bands are a shield that covers the whole body, physically, emotionally, mentally, and spiritually. It appears like an egg that surrounds us and vibrates various beautiful colors. When your aura is healthy, it will vibrate outward 2 to 3 feet. Some would call that our inner circle or our personal space. A weak or very ill person's auric field may only be 2 inches, and sometimes even less. Their aura will become weak and unstable or have darker colors. Our aura is the flow of life and connects our physical body with our spiritual body.

Chakra Energy: Chakras are swirling energy stations located down the center of our body. The word 'chakra' comes from Sanskrit and its translation is 'wheel' or 'disk.' Chakras are the spiritual energy centers within our body, the unseen, the store house of emotional events that have occurred in our lives. There are seven chakras, and each performs an energetic role. When I work with my own chakras, I like to run energy through them while meditating, which is like spinning a wheel in a clockwise direction in my mind's eye with both of my eyes closed. For the heart chakra, I sit with my eyes closed, concentrate on the heart chakra area, and imagine the wheels spinning down the left and up the right.

- Crown chakra: spirituality, consciousness, fulfillment, knowledge
- Third eye chakra: intuition, lucidity, meditation, trust
- Throat chakra: communication, expression, inspiration, creativity
- Heart chakra: love, healing, acceptance, compassion, sincerity
- Solar plexus chakra: wisdom, power, personality, strength, determination
- Sacral chakra: sexuality, sensuality, pleasure, sociability
- Root chakra: trust, energy, stability, comfort, safety

Look at the chakra descriptions. Pick one that you think you may need to work with. I work with the solar plexus a lot. I carry a lot of guilt and unworthiness in this area. How do I know that? Because my solar plexus is where I feel a sensation that I have named guilt. Anytime I worry, feel anxious, feel I messed something up, or blame myself, it causes my solar plexus to start to ache. The ache is on the inside of my body. I can press that area, and it bothers me. This sensation in my solar plexus also presents when I am having a hard time digesting things in my life. My career began to take a turn that was no longer in alignment with my beliefs and values. As I tried to make that job work, the pain in my solar plexus became a daily reminder that I was off track. As I was going through owning the practice, this spot would often act up. Patients' stories would get caught in that area and activate old scars of pain and mistrust. I could feel myself losing my power and not being the person I was truly meant to be.

While I focus on my solar plexus, I also know that working on the heart chakra helps me with self-love and self-acceptance. It took me five years to realize that the only way to correct that energy was to get into alignment with what I wanted and who I was meant to be.

Meridians: There are 12 main meridian lines that run energy throughout our bodies. Meridians move energy around the body like arteries move blood.

Meridians act as pathways that connect the energy centers or chakras in our body. Some explain meridians as our prana or life force. The meridian pathways are said to communicate information throughout the body and the mind. Meridians connect the emotions within the body to the physiology of the body. Think of stress and the chemicals stress makes. Stress doesn't just exist in our brain; it lives in all of our organs and tissues. The meridians can carry the coding of our emotions and be detected in acupuncture points located on our skin. The meridian system looks like a huge web that consists of a complex body map providing links and energy to all areas of our bodies.[15]

Energy Meridian Tapping: Tapping meridian and energy centers with the tips of your fingers balances your energy centers and can create a feeling of relaxation. Tapping techniques are numerous, but the one I want to spend time focusing on here are the three tapping centers that are easy to use anytime anywhere! I first learned about tapping from the Emotional Freedom Tapping work of Roger Callahan and Gary Craig. Their system includes scripts and nine different steps and tapping techniques.[16] I prefer the three meridian tapping points to teach patients a quick and easy process. The Three Tapping Points are being used by Seattle Children's Hospital. It distributes handouts to pediatric patients to explain tapping techniques, including The Three Tapping Points.[17] I love that a hospital is teaching kids how to calm themselves down and how to cope with stress and energy. This would be great for any of us and our patients.

The three points are the K27, the thymus, and the spleen. The K27 point is located an inch below the collar bone close to the sternum on each side. Tapping with the fingertips or rubbing the area on each side improves energy, alertness, and focus. After 30 seconds of tapping or rubbing, move to the thymus. It is located on the top half of our sternum. Again, tap or rub the area for 30 seconds. The thymus is considered the happiness center. If you only have time for one area, choose this one. It also will increase energy and strength. The third area is the spleen meridian. You will find this area located below the breast line on the ribs. The spleen meridian assists with energy and promotes immune function. This results in 1 1/2 minutes of tapping to restore energy, mood, and balance and boost the immune system. Voila! You can do this anywhere, anytime and teach anyone.

Running Healing Energy: We can also *run* healing energy through our body by using prayer and our hands. Our hands house our healing energy centers. Start by rubbing your hands together for a few seconds. Once they are warm, tap the center of each palm and say "on," then close your eyes and call in the white universal healing energy through the top of your head. Visualize this with your eyes closed, allowing the energy to go down your spine and through your body, out your feet. Then bring your hands to your forehead, the third eye, and point your fingers toward the third eye. Leave your hands there until you feel you are ready to move to the next chakra. Continue to move your hands down the different chakra systems while you pray and recite "letting go." You can learn more sophisticated techniques by studying *The Healing Code* by Dr. Alex Loyd. His technique is said to have healed Dr. Ben Johnson of Lou Gehrig's disease (ALS) in less than three months. Studies about the benefits of running healing energy have been conducted by Stanford, Harvard, Mayo Clinic, and the CDC.

~

The New Patient

She is a new patient, about 55 years old, who is here for back pain that has been ongoing for years. She has tried pain management, injections, pain medications, and physical therapy. She's seen a surgeon who told her she was not a surgery candidate. Nothing worked.

I sat with her. I took a deep breath and thought to myself, "I wonder what could possibly be causing this much pain." Through my years of spiritual work, I had learned a few things about energy. I felt driven to ask her if anything happened in her life that was painful or emotional. Her response was, "Yes, I was in a car accident in my twenties. My boyfriend and best friend were both killed."

Even though I hadn't known what to expect when I asked the question, I was not surprised that her pain was in her lumbar area—the root chakra. The root chakra is an area that indicates whether we feel safe and grounded in life. I took a deep breath and thought about all of this and tried to explain it to her the best I could without sounding cuckoo.

It was our first meeting in a modern, Western medicine clinic. She was not ready to hear about pain bodies and chakra systems, or that until she deals with the emotional trauma, the lumbar pain will never go away. Since all of the other approaches had not worked, I suggested it might be time to think outside the box.

In very small doses, I attempted to describe what I have learned about spirit and energy work. I recommended that she consider counseling, hypnosis, and energy work. I also gave her a referral to another surgeon and pain management specialist. I planted a seed of spiritual energy. What she does with it is up to her.

Nursing—Out of the Box

I think this is important for nurses and providers to know! Patients and providers have old wounds that many times have not been dealt with. We can lose our own energy providing patient care, which can be a source of burnout. Consider using the following techniques the next time you do an exam:

1. Look at your patient while holding positive thoughts and healing energy.

2. Every time you check the patient's heart, visualize that you are touching their heart chakra. Spin their wheel in your mind's eye, down the left, up the right. Spin yours, too!

3. For an abdominal exam, close your eyes and stop a moment over the solar plexus. Take a deep breath as you feel and listen to bowel sounds. (This is also a great time for you to breathe deeply and allow your relaxed energy to penetrate their energy.)

4. Be an energy force for your patient. As you breathe deeply, the patient will automatically mimic your breathing (see NLP, Chapter 4). You might tell your patient about breathing through their energy centers and allowing the natural healing energy to flow.

This practice of intentional breathing and focused energy is contrary to what is usually done when assessing patients. Usually, we are randomly thinking about all that we have to do. We are not really present. Our minds are racing at full throttle. Using this technique, you can slow your thoughts down for a nanosecond and just be with yourself and your patient.

Consider how you feel when you have a patient that is in terrible pain. You breathe faster and your energy changes. How about when they tell you about how they were abused as a child, how do you feel? The patient's negative energy is spilling onto you. I believe a lot of nurses and providers are naturally intuitive and can feel others' pains and emotions. Protect yourself by managing your energy and not absorbing theirs.

Every time you slow it down for your patient, you slow it down for yourself. If you are feeling rushed, anxious, or tired, observe how your patient reacts to you. Is your energy creating a rushed and anxious energy in them? Forget about running the quick exam just to get out of the room. Take time to breathe, visualize energy and touch the patient.

Touching the patients with purpose and pausing during the assessment is a connection so many providers gloss over. The actual touch of your hand, which is where much of your powerful healing energy is located, will transfer your energy to the patient. Make it good energy. Your energy can shift the vibration of the tissue that may need healing. If a patient is complaining of shoulder pain, linger with your hand on their shoulder, then take some deep breaths, ask questions, and do the assessment. Often patients will leave saying, "Huh, that feels better!" It's all about the provider setting the intention of healing.

Chapter Eight

Spirit Surrounds Us

We're no longer able to go through life on autopilot ...
we're being encouraged to wake up.
- Dr. Sue Morter

As I came in contact with more and more patients, one of the things I realized was that people are not just physical beings, but also spiritual beings. They don't go around talking about it, but it is in them. It is in you and me, too. As the years unfolded, I became more comfortable talking about spirit and asking questions about patients' beliefs.

If I had a stressed patient or one with a scary diagnosis, I often would soften my voice and ask them if they were spiritual. In 18 years, I cannot remember anyone ever saying they were not spiritual. This was an awakening for me. It's a conversation I rarely had with other people and then, at work, I was going there on a daily basis. As I started to ask patients if they were spiritual, the spiritual part of me began to grow.

Suddenly, I realized just how spiritual our world really is. We just don't stand up and start talking about it; it is very intimate. Every patient, every person, has an opinion on how to be present with spirit. When fears are high and emotions are out of control, I just slip in the kindest question of all, "Are you spiritual?" It's non-denominational and non-confrontational. It is a door that opens, allowing a deeper connection.

These connections and process of spirit are essential when we work with people. To become a more effective leader and healer, I learned my focus could not just be on the physical symptoms that bring the client in. In fact, the physical often masks something much deeper. Finding a way to address that deeper thing with patients brings a kind of relaxation and openness to the patients. Once I approached the subject by asking if they were spiritual, many patients opened up and often shared their beliefs, telling me they know that God (however defined) hears their prayers.

Many people do not realize there are no mistakes. I believe everything in life is divinely orchestrated, that we are a work in progress here to learn lessons to become better spirits. I think as we mature, we realize the spiritual aspects of life are real and present, but we have to seek spirituality to really get to know it. It is also my belief that we are all divinely interconnected and need to be open to the power of what is showing up in our lives and ask why.

I believe that if you are reading this book, it was because you were meant to.

You must somehow have needed it.

I also believe that we are all put into each other's lives for a reason and season. That includes the patients that are put on our paths, as well. Some patients irritate something inside of ourselves while others remind us of how divine we are.

We have what they need, or they have what we need in the way of growth and lessons. Either we are here to help them, or they are here to help us. Whether we know it or not, we are all impacting each other. We need to open ourselves and invite spiritual awareness.

The Door that Opens

I love what spirit has to offer me at work. Often, patients will bring Bibles or some other spiritual text, holding their books on their lap. I have had patients ask if they could pray for me, and I took that as a sign that I could ask if I could pray for them, when appropriate. It is magical to sit with a patient and pray. The room is quiet, we take a deep breath, relax, the emotions are calmed, and the connection to the Divine is present.

Being open to questions and answers about faith and spirituality provides even more tools to help patients heal and connect with their health care team.

Prayer is powerful.

A Course in Miracles

I was shopping at Goodwill. I love books and always browse the titles there. I saw two books on the shelf entitled *A Course in Miracles* and thought, "I want miracles," so I purchased them. They had a home on my shelf. I would open one and think "wow, that's deep" and then put it back on the shelf. Years went by and one day I was listening to a podcast by Marianne Williamson speaking about love and ego. She referenced *A Course in Miracles* throughout her talk and I thought, "Do I have those books?" I looked on my shelf, found them, committed to the daily mantras, and took my first step into the journey of self-discovery, of learning that I am a spiritual being living in ego or living in love.

A Course in Miracles (ACIM) was written by Helen Schucman to be a guide to spiritual enlightenment. The theme is to gain awareness of how love is present in our lives. The lessons guide the student's mind from "condemnation out of fear" to "forgiveness out of love." There are 365 days of affirmations that help anyone looking to transform their life from the fear the ego imagines to true love of source.

Meditating on the affirmations every day, I was able to rewire my brain to new attitudes and ideas. I credit those books to my success at reducing my fear and ego-driven ideas and entering a state of love through forgiveness. At a slow pace, the spirit of those books began to teach me to love, and to let go of fear and anxiety. Over the years,

I have always kept the books close. I like to write down the lessons on index cards, then repeat them over and over during the day, e.g., *God is in everything I see because God is in me.* For the last 41 days, I have been back into the book every day. This is my fourth time doing the daily work. I have only made it through the year once. Today my lesson is, *God goes with me wherever I go.* The premise is that I am a spiritual being and that I am not alone; God is always with me. All day today, I will read that lesson from my index card and crowd out any negativity that tries to sneak in and steal my joy.

I have done the lessons on and off so many times that certain lessons have become ingrained in my brain. I often find those index cards in strange places: the laundry, glove box, pockets of my jackets, the bottom of my purse. I smile when I find a card, read it, and safely tuck it back in its hiding place for next time. I am a huge fan.

How can ACIM help you? If you want to find a way to stop judging yourself and others, try ACIM. If you want to get rid of fear, ACIM will help you find peace and love. If you want to become at peace with your life journey and release negative self-talk and anxiety, try ACIM. If you want to be more spiritual and help more people, learn ACIM. Even if you don't do it every day, doing it once brings you closer to sanity.

The Law of Attraction

The first time I heard about Esther Hicks, also known as Abraham Hicks, I thought, "Wow! Is that real?" Again, like ACIM, I didn't listen the first time I was introduced to her work. But as spirit will have its way, it kept creeping into my life until I took a good look at it.

I went to the library and checked out her book, *The Law of Attraction: The Basics of the Teachings of Abraham,* 2006. Once I began reading, I immediately was drawn into the teachings. Spirit is simple; we make it complicated.

Whether or not you believe that we are spiritual beings having a human experience, the book clearly defines a philosophy of love that no one can deny. We are here to enjoy our life, to live a life fulfilled. When you begin to practice Abraham's teaching, it makes so much sense. We create the disconnection from spirit by never getting into it. We decide not to pursue our spiritual care by not engaging in it.

The *Law of Attraction,* according to Abraham, requires four steps: Ask for what you want. Send a signal or vibration.

- Source answers. There is a time gap; be okay with that. It comes in a vibrational form first.

- Feel that it is already done. Receive without the evidence. You allow it. Believe.

- Attitude of appreciation. Draw in what you want by saying thank you before you receive it.

Remember to eliminate scarcity barriers. Avoid thinking that there will not be enough. If you ask to receive more money and yet you still feel broke, you are not in alignment with spirit. Your vibrational alignment is incongruent. You are living in lack instead of abundance.

Today I listened to one of the YouTube teachings by Abraham. It was all about starting the first 17 seconds of your day in spirit. Instead of waking up and saying, "I don't want to get up," or "Jeez, I don't want to go to work," think loving thoughts:

"I am connected to source, and I love living in this world."

"I wonder what miracle awaits me today."

I utilize the first breath of the morning to optimize positivity and gratitude. This sends a vibration into the day that you are open and willing to receive.

I love thinking about creating a better future. I've spent most of my life reliving the past, reflecting on what happened yesterday, how I got this way, what I could have done differently to have a different outcome. Now, I am concentrating on my God-given right to happiness.

In modern medicine, drugs became the go-to for health. As medication became such a potent release of patients' symptoms, we stopped needing spirit. But spirit is always within us, we cannot deny it. A day will come when each of us will search for meaning in our own lives. I recommend starting by watching a few videos of Abraham Hicks and listening for your truths.

Can Spirituality be Detected in the Brain?

Studies have been done to see if the brain has a spiritual neuronal connection. According to researchers, spiritual experiences involve "pronounced shifts in perception [that] buffer the effects of stress.[18] The findings suggest that those experiences can be accessed by everyone. They noted the neural correlation of spirituality and the comforting centers in the brain. A range of specific neural structures in the brain have been linked to spirituality and religion.[19]

Prayer Circles

My grandmother was a very faithful woman. She kept her tattered Bible beside her chair. She was hoping to live to 100, but in her late nineties, she fell in the bathroom, hit her head, and couldn't get up. She dragged her painful, bleeding body from the back of her house to the front of her house, and somehow pulled herself onto her front porch. She weakly called for help. As spirit would have it, a neighbor was out for a walk, heard her small voice, and called the ambulance. The emergency room doctor told my aunt to call the family because she wasn't going to make it. Her heart rate was exceptionally low and her blood pressure barely audible.

We all rushed to the hospital. As we stood there feeling helpless, we thought, "What would Grandma do?" Then we circled her bed, held hands and prayed, silently standing and asking God to help her as tears rolled down our cheeks.

That moment touched us all. I believe that every person in my family implanted that prayerful moment in their hearts. It was beautiful and serene. I felt I was part of something bigger, the love of the universe.

An hour later, as we were waiting for her to pass, her pulse and blood pressure began to change. She began to pump back to life. For me, the experience was rich with family, love, and spirit. I know for that moment in time, we were all connected, and we were one. We all felt it.

Compassionate Actions

Loving and spirit go together. Nurses are loving spirits. Some days are better than others, but we always enter the work with an open heart of compassion. As nurses, we can help others be compassionate, too. We can help by putting a 'do not disturb' sign on the door to keep visitors out after a hard night or telling the rounding doctors to go to that room last. Small things. Most often, it's small things, like the smile that comes when the curtains are pulled back and the light flows into the room.

Spirit Leaders

I started working with spirit leaders to help strengthen my connection with God. What I found out was that there are people all over the world praying for all of us. When I learned Pranic Healing, I learned the prayer of Grand Master Choa Kok Sui. He emphasizes in his practice that we are all brought together to do "meditation and spiritual work to heal humanity and our planet." I bought his audio prayer and meditation. It is so healing. Until I did Pranic Healing, I never did a concentrated prayer for 'our' world. Now I see the implications of helping other people, using prayer to connect us all as one. All over the world Pranic practitioners meet once a month to pray and do healing work for our entire universe. We are spirit, we are healers.

I met a beautiful soul named Beth who was doing healing energy work. She traveled to Peru to become a shaman and became open to conversation with Jesus. I set up an appointment to meet her and had several awesome sessions with her. Her home has many sacred spaces and altars that are very spiritual. She told me that she participates in universal healing. She is a part of a group of people in different parts of the world who pray at the same time for healing for our planet. Isn't that awesome?

I also have been doing one-on-one sessions with Gina Nicole for years. I took her certification class on tarot, and she has been my mentor ever since. She is a great guide in my spiritual practices. She knows a lot of the spiritual leaders in St. Louis, and she often does Zoom calls with them to help healers have their voices heard.

I hope this gives you an idea about how much is going on around you. There are people everywhere that are helping us spiritually. You can find people in your own hometown simply by attending a class at one of the spiritual stores. I Googled 'spiritual stores in St. Louis' and found a variety of different places. Once you go and meet people, you will begin to crave continued enlightenment.

Ho'oponopono Healing Process

At age 67, Morrnah Simeona introduced the Ho'oponopono healing process at the Huna World Convention in Punalu'u, Hawaii.

I first learned about it in a class I took at a store called Silver Lining. Gina Nicole taught us the practice of Ho'oponopono. She explained how our pains are inside of us and we need to do forgiveness work to release them. Our fears, insecurities, and guilt are alive from long ago. Ho'oponopono is about forgiving the pain that we created inside of us and learning to love ourselves.

I did the Ho'oponopono work to release guilt and shame within myself. I hold guilt and unworthiness inside my solar plexus chakra, right beneath my ribs in the center of my chest. Guilt and unworthiness have been my lifelong companions, especially during trying times. That's why my forgiveness work is on childhood traumas.

One of the experiences that traumatized me was when I was 16 years old working at McDonald's. A man drove into the parking lot after closing and pulled out a gun. He was a big man, and it was a long gun. He pointed the gun at my head and said, "Someone is going to let me into the safe or I am going to blow this little lady's head off." At once, I began to scream and freak out. Long story short, he went on to rob our store and left eight of us in a closet. I thought I was going to die. I was so traumatized.

That experience has given me fear, panic, and anxiety. No one would expect anything different. The problem is that I am 57 years old now and when I feel threatened or like someone is coming after me, I can feel my heart race, my breath stop, and I want to run for my life. It is a response to an old memory. Why do I keep putting myself through those emotions? Because they are stored in my brain and DNA.

Applying the Ho'oponopono will clean those memories and replace them with love. When I apply Ho'oponopono, I take responsibility for my own thoughts and feelings. The gunman is not currently creating the feelings of fear inside of me. I am. I take 100% responsibility for creating the pain within me, and now I can begin to do the cleaning work. Cleaning work is continuous because there always will be feelings that we create from some dysfunction in our lives. Cleaning involves repeating the verses of Ho'oponopono.

I'm sorry. Please forgive me. Thank you. I love you.

I use the Ho'oponopono verses to release the pain within me and then forgive myself for hurting myself. It is powerful. Then I add in breathing exercises. I like to breathe in "I'm sorry," hold the breath to "please forgive me," blow out to "thank you," and hold the breath to "I love you."

The insight is that all of the pain is stored within us so we can heal ourselves and the universe by using forgiveness and love. It becomes a spiritual relationship.

The main purpose of this process is to discover the Divinity within oneself. The Ho'oponopono is a profound gift which allows one to develop a working relationship with the Divinity within and learn to ask that in each moment, our errors in thought, word, deed or action be cleansed. The process is essentially about freedom, complete freedom from the past. – Morrnah Nalamaku Simeona

Our Calling is a Gift

As nurses we don't always recognize the precious gift we have in our calling to help others. Most of us don't understand that we actually came into this world to be nurses to care for people in all different walks of life. We decided on our calling, or when the call came, we answered. It is a blessing and sometimes a curse. I get afraid I am going to fail, hurt someone, say something wrong, prescribe the wrong therapy or forget to order the right test.

But now I am learning that each day is a gift. I pray in the morning for God to send whoever needs me and to help me provide what they need. I use prayer to help me move into the next level of spirituality. I am able to help more people when I am living in spirit because I see, hear, feel all of the spiritual gifts that God has bestowed on me.

As humans, each of us has these gifts. Learning to connect to them can help reduce the stress in our days. The spirit will help us breathe life in and let anxiety go. And the best part is we can begin to believe in it enough to tell other people about it. I believe in HOPE: Helping Other People Everywhere. Open your heart, have optimism, pause in your life and see the beauty, and energize your goals.

Both of these messages reflect my calling. We must each decide on our own.

Here is a great spirit story:

I was getting ready to do spiritual hypnosis with Debbie. We had talked about spiritual hypnosis and what she hoped to achieve by doing it. I had my tarot card deck sitting on the table with my essential oils. I forgot my pen, so I left to go get it. When I came back, we started with a prayer for guidance to our session.

Then I asked her to give me a number between 1 and 10. She picked 5. I shuffled my tarot deck five times. I pulled out a card that would help guide our hypnosis session that day. As I pulled it out, her mouth opened wide, and her eyes got big.

I said, "What's the matter?"

She excitedly admitted, "While you were out of the room, I pulled a card out of your deck, and it is the exact same card you just pulled."

Spirit is always with us. She was pleasantly surprised, and I smiled really big, thanking the universe.

Spiritually, we are all connected to the universe and can tap into that source with persistence and patience. When you are in spirit you realize that everything you do matters and touches lives. You become the one who challenges the fear and ego and offers up love and acceptance. This becomes a fulfillment of one's truest path of life.

Spirit is working all around us if we are open and invite it in. There are special moments in our lives when we are awakened, when other people teach us and impregnate us with spirit. It is a process that takes time, just like planting a seed and fertilizing it again and again and again.

Spirit is the breath of life, the feeling of belonging to something bigger than ourselves. It is not something we have to talk about. It just is. However, we have to do the work to bring the spirit in. That spirit will create a sense of peace within us and a total acceptance that others' issues are not about us. Let them keep their junk. Stay present and be peaceful. No one can steal our peace. We decide if we want to give it away.

Here are few things we can do to help ourselves:

- Stay present.
- Practice Ho'oponopono when feeling anxious or angry.
- Practice forgiveness work.
- Get and use ACIM and decide that you want to be free from the insanity that is called life and contain the reality that is called spirit and love.
- Ask patients, "Are you spiritual?"
- Ask yourself if you're living in ego or in love.
- Align with the Law of Attraction. Learn how to call your day in.

Chapter Nine

Finding the Calm:
Brain Waves and Meditation

Your goal is not to battle with the mind, but to witness the mind.
— Swami Muktananda

I have a high-strung personality that has no release button. When my kids started to go off to high school and college, they didn't need me anymore. I had been their soccer coach, volleyball coach, and room mom. When that stopped, I started going to Toastmasters, trying out Functional Medicine seminars and increasing my work hours. I'll be damned if I was going to slow down. I ignored the need to slow down and kept charging ahead. I bought a medical practice and joined groups of masterminds.

Unfortunately, with each thing I added, I began to feel more and more heaviness inside. I loved everything I was doing, but it was taking a toll on my body and my life. How did I know? I began to feel racy inside, I couldn't fall asleep at night, I had a lot of negative thoughts, I stopped going out with friends, and I never felt peaceful. I was in constant motion jumping from one thing to the next.

I was able to handle the stress for a long time, but eventually the bombs kept getting bigger and more frequent. I needed a calming solution to my overcompensating lifestyle before I was headed for a breakdown or disease.

The stress of a busy life leaves the brain with an electrical shortage. I was definitely feeling this. I learned about meditation but didn't quite understand how it could help me.

Then I arrived at a place in my life where the stress was bigger than me. I wanted to give up. What could I do to help myself learn to relax? That's when I found relief through a movie. I watched *The War Room* and became intrigued.

I really connected with the movie. It was about an older woman who was selling her house. When she showed the realtor the 'war room,' the realtor became very inquisitive. The older woman told her the closet was her sacred space for prayer. She would hang her prayers on the walls and sit in peacefulness with the Lord.

My biggest take away from that movie was to build my own war room. My husband had built a closet in the basement for extra storage. After the movie, I took over the closet. I put the rocking chair I used to rock my kids in when they were little inside. I added a small folding table and put framed pictures of Jesus, Mother Mary, Archangel Michael and Archangel Gabrielle on it. I put candles that flicker in the darkness, providing the perfect amount of light.

It's where I go every morning. I hang words of prayers on the walls, I hang motivational phrases, I have essential oils and holy water. My Bible and A Course in Miracles (ACIM) sit by my side. I keep a handful of index cards to write my daily scripture or ACIM mantra. I love this space. I share it with blankets and clothes that are hanging up around me. When that door closes, it's Donna time. Do not disturb me. I sit there anywhere from 30 minutes to an hour in meditation, trying to slow my brainwaves and receive the peace of God.

Over the last five years, this has been my sanctuary. I never would have made it through the crisis of my emotional and stressful life without it. I clean all my worry in there, I breathe in the light of healing, I close my mind to the swirling thoughts. I create mind movies of my future. That movie was a God intervention for sure. The room is my sanity.

Meditation

When I do things, I always want to know why. I ask how meditating can really help me. In my research about how meditation was going to help me, I discovered how many influential people practice it. Then I looked into the studies to see if there was any proof that meditation really helped people heal. I was pleasantly surprised by how much literature there was to support meditation as a health and wellness practice. The studies report that meditation calms the brain and teaches the neurons to rest and correct.

Many successful people meditate: Jerry Seinfeld, Madonna, Hugh Jackman, Lady Gaga, Oprah and more. All of them would tell you that meditation is a necessary tool for survival in the fast lane. It adds to our creativity and allows us to have peace in our busy worlds. It is a spiritual connection as well.

Meditation stops the excessive worry, stops the repetitive mind race, and causes us to try to live in the here and now. The trick to meditation is to just start with five minutes. Sitting for too long is not easy at first; our minds and emotions can get frantic. It's best to do it first thing in the morning when brain vibrations aren't in full throttle. Meditation is about learning to discipline our brains. It's about settling down the brain one electron at a time. Turning the system off.

The dangers of always staying busy and never allowing time to reflect and be peaceful results in a stressed-out life. And stress does not come by itself. It invites inflammation that increases the likelihood of disease. It encourages divorces and dwells on dissatisfaction. The stressed brain is like a spoiled child having a tantrum to get what he wants.

Brain Waves[20]

The brain is made up of electrical waves. The electroencephalo-gram (EEG) is a measurement of wavelengths in our brains. Basically, the EEG captures the electrical activity of the functioning brain.

The brain wavelengths are: gamma, beta, alpha, theta, delta. Each of these waves represents a different state of consciousness. Gamma brain waves are the highest speed waves. We use gamma brain waves when we are concentrating hard on something, in deep thought or problem solving.

As adults, we spend most of our awake time with our brains in a high beta brain wave. We live in this wave throughout the day with brief drifts into alpha states. Beta brain waves can become relentless and cause stress if we do not learn how to shut down the chatter of the inner critic.

We drift into alpha when we are relaxed. We are also in alpha when we first wake up in the morning and as we begin to fall asleep. When our brains are in the alpha state, we are not totally conscious and can receive relaxation messages. This makes morning and evening the optimal time to perform meditation.

Theta is the brain wave of deep meditation or light sleep. It is in the cusp of going from alpha to theta that the magic happens in the brain. Theta is all about dreaming, learning, and intuition.

Delta brain waves are our slowest brain waves, and this is where deep sleep occurs. Some people who practice transcendental medita-tion can enter delta brain waves and make deep connections. This is called 'total detachment.'

Knowing about the different states of brain waves and learning techniques can help us take ourselves out of crazy beta and into calm-ing alpha or theta.

Meditation is one way, breath work is another; anything that can turn down the signals in the brain to help it relax. The beauty of this is that we can teach our brains how to relax. We tell ourselves, "This is how we do it. Meditate, breathe, stop, rest, and reset."

When beta kicks into automatic, our brains can get locked. Then in the evening, fatigued from convoluted thinking, we enter the alpha state, most likely in front of a television as we download messages about delicious burgers and fries. We could be using that alpha time to become peaceful and relaxed.

Children and their Brain Waves

Interestingly, data suggests children are born in the delta wave and stay there until they are 2 years old. Think of them as chronically asleep. When children are between the ages of 2 and 6, they are in theta waves, the most imaginative, living primarily in their inner state. They have not conformed to the world. They daydream and are super charged to learn, not to rationalize. Then, between ages 5 and 8, they begin to have more alpha waves. They are interpreting and drawing conclusions about life; however, their imaginative inner world is still very active. After turning 8 years old, they slowly begin to join the conscious world and add on beta waves. Their conscious minds become awakened.

What's important about all of this? This crucial brain development time is a perfect window of opportunity to mold our children's future for love and success. We want to help "pave the wave" for children before they become adults. This is a rich time to emphasize the importance of coping strategies, meditation, prayer, love, security, and critical thinking skills. We, as teachers, parents, and providers, need to provide them with the tools that can help them meet and love themselves. We want to help them defend against negative programming. Any of us who work with children can teach them about brain waves and help them learn how to be more in control of their emerging 'consciousness.' Once we are adults, the programs are written, and it becomes much more difficult to change our minds about our lives.

Meditation is on the Rise[21]

In a National Health survey, it was found that in the U.S., adults' use of meditation in the past 12 months tripled between 2012 and 2017 (from 4.1% to 14.2%). The use of meditation by children in this country also increased significantly (from 0.6 % in 2012 to 5.4 % in 2017).[22]

This is a significant improvement and a sign that people are becoming enlightened to the Universal Laws of the mind and spirit. The mind and the spirit are one, and meditation is what makes that so.

Research on Nothingness

It is genuinely difficult for humans to sit and be quiet. Researcher Timothy Wilson of the University of Virginia conducted a study that confirms how crazy we can become when left alone with our own thoughts.

The researchers took a group of adults and told them that the study was about sitting alone doing nothing. Each participant was hooked up to a machine that was capable of giving them an electrical jolt. Each participant was given one jolt before the study period to experience the sensation. Some of the participants said that they would pay money to never feel that kind of shock again, and yet, 25% of the women and approximately 66% of the men shocked themselves when they were left alone. One person zapped himself 190 times in the 15-minute block.[23]

This study provides us with feedback about how difficult it is to sit and do nothing. If it is difficult to be alone and do nothing, imagine our patients, sitting in our waiting rooms, potentially with stress and uncertainty churning around in their heads.

Benefits of Meditation[24]

Meditation improves different functions of the brain. Harvard University conducted a study that showed meditation leads to thicker gray matter in the areas of the brain that are responsible for our feelings of compassion and self-awareness. It also documented that during meditation, the frontal lobe of the brain stops trying to analyze and lets the body relax. The thalamus, which is our relay station in the brain, slows down and allows us to feel calm.

It is believed that anxiety is formed from numerous neural pathways located in the medial prefrontal cortex of the brain, the area connected to fear.

Meditation affects these pathways, allowing for the reduction of anxiety.

Alpha waves are boosted by meditation practices because of the release of serotonin, which can reduce stress levels and improve memory. According to Jill Goldstein, a professor of psychiatry and medicine at Harvard Medical School, stress affects not only memory but many other brain functions, including mood and anxiety, as well as promotes inflammation, which adversely affects our health.

Studies done at Wisconsin-Madison University showed that meditation helps the amygdala recover more quickly from stress and trauma. Creativity improves with meditation. Meditation research done by Osher Research Center found that people who performed mindful meditation could change the brain waves and tune out distractions. These changes increased study participants' productivity and boosted memory.

Transcendental Meditation (TM®) practitioners did a five-year study published in 2012 on patients with known coronary heart disease. The group who used transcendental meditation were reported to be 48% less likely to die of a heart attack or stroke than subjects in the control group. Their research further found that TM® practice is "clinically meaningful" in regard to its potential to decrease systolic and diastolic blood pressure.[25]

Teaching Yourself to Meditate

When you begin to meditate, consider the following:

- The timing of your meditation is very important. It is best to start meditation first thing in the morning and/ or before bed. This is the time you are most likely to be in the alpha state.

- It is important to sit up when you meditate with your back straight. Lying in bed will encourage sleep.

- If you are new to it, start with 5 minutes or less. You can set a timer on your phone.

- Keep on trying; never give up. This is for you. For your health. For your well-being. For your calmness. For your sanity. For your life training. For connecting with source.

- Make it a routine. Do it at the same time, in the same way, at the same place every day. Enjoy it.

- Practice using your meditation to color your world. Visit the Akashic records, symbolically journey with shamanic travel, sit silently or fly high. Use a movie projector to see yourself in the future or rest in mindfulness and find peace. Breathe through your heart and find love. Pull in colors of the chakra world. Pray and dance with the spirit of your choice. Think of it as a time to play out your dreams and inspirations. Use imagination to create the world you really want. Any dream is possible if you set it free. Explore the beautiful world of your mind. Imagine drawing a picture of your future, then sitting in it and experiencing it as if it already has happened. The brain does not know the difference between reality and imagination. So, once you imagine it, the brain will get to work to make it happen.

Neurons that Wire Together Fire Together

I can't repeat this too often: neurons that wire together fire together. Brains do this through repetitive firing of learned neurons. When you meditate, you enter the alpha state to imagine and dream, which means new neurons are firing. Your brain is learning and making new connections.

There are many types of meditation techniques. Explore. Find those that work for you, so your brain can keep learning and connecting.

Practice, Practice, Practice

Exercise improves our physical performance. Exercising the brain is the same, and one of the best exercises for the brain is meditation. For it to work, we need to practice it daily. Meditation helps stop negative thought patterns and burn in new positive patterns. It helps remove emotions that no longer serve us and embeds positive reinforcements for what we want to believe and how we want to behave.

If we practice our meditation every day, eventually we will be able to reduce our stress. Then, when we feel stress during the day (beta waves gone wild), we will be able to enter relaxation easily on a command breath and rest (alpha waves). We must first be consciously aware that the beta waves have gone mad, then we must respond by using relaxation techniques. This is the point of meditation. I am not sure why meditation has gotten such a woo woo name. The results are undeniable, as is the research.

Patient Story

I have a patient who is 67 years old. She came in to get cigarette counseling because of her severe chronic lung disease. Her pulmonologist told her if she didn't quit, she would die in the next two years. I asked her if she had any issues with depression. She told me she had been depressed her whole life. I asked her to tell me a little about her depression and she said, "Oh, it's much better now. I got so bad a few years ago I didn't think I could go on. I had become very suicidal. My counselor introduced me to meditation, and it has been the only thing that has ever helped my depression." I asked about her meditation rituals. She said she uses transcendental meditation twice a day and that she could not live without it.

She seemed like an unlikely user of meditation, but she affirmed for me the importance of how much the practice can change brain chemistry and help people cope better with life.

To find the right practice and insights for you to calm your mind, explore and practice the following:

A Course In Miracles: Every day for one year, read through *A Course In Miracles*. Learn to do a mantra every day and meditate on it. This requires mind searching and is different from sitting quietly.

This work brings me great peace through resisting the ego energy of fear and pain and replacing it with love and spirit.

Loving Kindness Meditation: Focus on your heart during this meditation. Remember people and things you love. Send love into the universe—to everyone or anyone. Then draw the love back into yourself and hold onto that love; you are worthy.

Transcendental Meditation: You have to take classes and learn from a registered provider.

Mindful Meditation: Stay present; concentrate on the breath and try to slow the brain down. Be quiet and consistent, refocusing on your breath. You can be mindful anywhere. When you are feeling stressed at work, try looking at your hand, the lines on your hand. Are they big or small? Can you count them? What color is your palm? Squeeze your hand shut three times and open it. Is it any different? You have just taken your mind off of whatever is bothering you.

Guided/Unguided Meditations: There are many to pick from; look them up online. The practice of binaural beats using headphones allows the brain to create a third beat from the two different beats it hears. The third beat is calming and relaxing.

Drumming: Used by shamans to meet your spirit guide.

Akashic Records: A place you can go in meditation to review your books and records of your life.

Chapter Ten

Spirit is in the Breath and the Breath is in Us

Breathing in, I center myself, breathing out I smile.
-Thich Nhat Hanh

We breathe different kinds of breaths. There is the short anxiety breath, the sigh breath and the deep breath. Sometimes we even forget to breathe, exhibiting short, shallow breaths that are tight and full of anxiety. The breath is the cleansing of carbon dioxide and the refueling of oxygen. Every cell of our bodies relies on the work of our breath.

A single breath, if done right, can change our physiology. Many people suck at breathing. I know that sounds strange, but let's face it, most people do not breathe purposefully. We take our breath for granted. Many people breathe hunching over a computer or lying on a sofa. When our body is in a weak position, you lose the full exhalation mechanism. When we hunch over or take a short breath, we only exhale 70% of the carbon dioxide in our lungs. Not optimal gas exchange!

Right now, sit up straight or stand up tall, take a big breath, and blow it all out. As a matter of fact, blow it out some more, really exhaling all of the contents of the lungs as you pull up the diaphragm into your chest cavity. How does that feel?

Breath work is central to mind, body, and emotional health. As nurses and providers, we need to understand that the simple act of deep breathing releases the vagal response and recruits calming of the parasympathetic nervous system. Also, the act of breathing synchronizes our brain waves, heart beats, and respiratory rates.

We breathe between 12 to 20 breaths a minute, or between 17,000 to 30,000 breaths a day. It is said that to increase our life span, we must reduce our regular respiratory rate from 16 breaths a minute to 10. This can be done through concentrated, purposeful breathing.

Simply sit and take three deep breaths very slowly—in for five, hold for five, out for five, hold for five, then do it over again.

In nursing school, we learn to tell people to take a deep breath and cough, but I had no idea the implications of breath work until I began to study it deeper. We all know as nurses that, after surgery, using an incentive spirometer reduces the risk of pneumonia, but I rarely see those patients take the spirometer home with them. It's a shame really, especially when you know that the incentive spirometer allows more air to inflate the lungs and open airways to prevent fluid and mucus buildup. It is definitely a good exercise for sick patients. I am sure it would also help recovering patients, too.

Diaphragmatic breathing, or deep breathing, is breathing that is done by contracting the diaphragm, a muscle located horizontally between the thoracic cavity and abdominal cavity. Air enters the lungs, you allow the belly to expand instead of the chest. Using our diaphragm to breathe instead of our chest allows the body to trade more incoming oxygen for outgoing carbon dioxide, causing the heart rate to slow down and lower the blood pressure.

Exemplifying the "learn one, teach one" philosophy presented earlier, Johns Hopkins Hospital is teaching this technique to children and adults for stress and pain management. We have to start trying to get these techniques in the EMRs as handouts for patients to take home.

Can our respiratory rate change our physiology? Findings from the National Institutes of Health (NIH) "revealed that sick people are more inclined to have respiratory rate variability patterns. In the study, respiratory rate had a high indicator of deteriorating health." [26]

Breathe and Let Go

The question I want us to address is, "What if we worked better to help ourselves and our patients control our breathing while relaxing into a minute or two of mindfulness?"

Mindfulness is that moment you take to just be. Simply put, you sense your surroundings, you take in what you visualize around you, you appreciate the air that is coming into your lungs, you feel your body relax and just be. How would a simple command to a patient to just breathe and let go make a difference? When I have a patient that comes in and they are clearly a mess, I tell them to stop and breathe. I show them a few breathing exercises and watch the magic happen.

I like to educate patients about the benefits of breathing through their stress response. I tell them that when they are stressed and worrying, they are producing inflammation, and that inflammation can cause disease and disruption in their bodies.

So, what can we do differently for our patients? Once we understand the benefits of various types of stress management techniques, we can introduce them to other people. Imagine our kids, our spouses, and our patients being able to slow down and be present, and just breathe instead of living in the frenzy of the world.

What if you put together a handout for patients and asked your employer if you could scan it into the EMR? I love this idea.

The Doorknob or S.T.O.P. Practice[27]

The S.T.O.P. Practice helps lower blood pressure, reduce anxiety, decrease pain, lower symptoms of depression, and improve sleep. Use it when you are feeling you need to stop and breathe. It starts by attempting to pull ourselves out of autopilot mode. Next, you want to see with clarity, and practice being present.

S. Stop what you're doing.

T. Take a few breaths.

O. Observe and check in with what's going on within you.

P. Pick how to proceed. Ask yourself, "What is the most beneficial thing to do next?"

In medicine, it's often called a doorknob practice because it only takes a few moments. Each time you put your hand on a doorknob to enter a room for the next interaction with another human being, whether it is a patient visit or an administrative meeting, you can: *Stop. Take a few breaths. Observe and notice how things are. Pick how to proceed with intention.*

Breath Work Options:[28]

- Alternative Nostril Breath Work: Use your right hand and plug your left nostril with your pointer finger while breathing in your right nostril. Then plug off your right nostril with your thumb and breathe out through your left nostril. Then breathe in through your left nostril, then out your right nostril while plugging as above.

- Diaphragmatic Breathing: Stand up, fold your hands together behind your head, breathe in through your nose and out your mouth, then raise your arms. This stabilizes the chest muscles and makes you use the diaphragm. Watch your belly rise and fall. Practice. I like the breath of counting in for five, hold for five, out for five, hold for five. This slows you down and allows you to enter alpha states.

- Lay on the bed and put your hand on your belly. Breathe in through your nose and out through your mouth. You want your hand to rise when you breathe in and sink the abdomen when you breathe out. This breath exercise can calm our nerves, reduce cortisol excitability, and reduce our stress response.

- The Breath of Fire: This is truly my favorite. With this breath, you breathe in and out through your nose and try to count up to 30 with very quick breaths. When you get done, your head is spinning and feels great.

- Squeeze and Hold Breath Work: I love this one too. Start by squeezing your hands and feet, arms and legs, your abdomen and chest, and then slowly squeeze your whole body and hold your breath. Once you breathe and release, you feel great. Wiggle your hands, and let the energy run out.

- Heart Breath Work: Teach patients to breathe through their heart, first by placing their hand over their heart and then breathing in five breaths through the nose, hold five breaths while thinking loving thoughts, take five breaths out through the mouth, finishing with a swoosh, and hold five breaths.

- Spirit Breath Work: Feel the universe filling you with air as you inhale. Allow the life force to flow through you. Sense the space of this energy within yourself. Notice how this energy connects you with a deeper part of yourself. As you exhale, send the energy to all living things around you.

When I do breath work, I imagine a white light all around me, coming in through the top of my head into my whole body.

Chapter Eleven

The Stories We Tell Ourselves

An old person dies ... a book is lost.
- Slim and Thompson, 1985

Stories have the power to make us or break us. I first learned about stories through Toastmasters. I would weave a story and end with a powerful punch line to woo my audience. I had a great coach, Kristen. She made everyone in our group tell their story until they could tell it in short sentences and still make an impact.

My story is the one that created my vision of who I am becoming and why I want to be that woman.

My story started with desertion, lived through trauma, developed an engine of anxiety, powered up the brain, trained to survive, and began to fight a good fight.

I suffered many traumas in my younger years. The pain drove me to find solutions to become healthier and happier. Because I have done the work to improve my disposition, I am able to help others journey more confidently through their stories. Our story is what we live by and who we become. Our stories tell others our perception of life, so choose wisely.

My First Story Cycle

One of my earliest memories is when my father left me when I was 5 years old. My parents were divorced, and I was visiting my dad. I wasn't allowed to stay at his house, so I was at my grandparent's house. He promised to come by in the morning to see me, but the only thing he left was a goodbye letter. In it, he told my grandparents that he had packed up my other siblings and left for California.

Hysteria ensued. I couldn't stop crying and screaming for my dad. My poor grandparents were besides themselves. They had just found out that their son and grandchildren were gone, and now his other daughter was having an emotional meltdown.

My aunt came and drove me home. For 45 minutes, I knelt in the backseat, staring out the back window, watching every set of head-lights. I was so sure my father was behind us, racing to come get me. With each passing mile, I realized he wasn't coming.

Over the years, my expectations about my dad changed, and our connection faded. I learned to accept that he would promise to visit, but those visits would never happen.

When I was 21 years old, he moved back to St. Louis. I decided it was time for me to air my resentment so I could feel better. I called him and invited him out for pizza and beer. Finally, after all those years, I was able to tell my dad how I felt. "You were such a bad dad," I told him. I talked about all of the times he disappointed me. I was such a little girl, and I didn't understand why he left me behind.

He didn't interrupt, and he never got angry at my accusations. Instead, he listened. Then he proceeded to tell his side of the story; one I had never thought about before.

His own father was an alcoholic. Some of his earliest memories were of loud bars and late nights. Growing up, he never quite lived up to his father's expectations, and he always came in second to his wildly successful brother.

He told me of how limited his access was to me, that my mother was afraid he'd take me from her. He had asked her to send me to California for a visit, but my mom refused. Back then, once a child went over state lines, a father could keep her and the mother would have no rights.

I realized that my father had abandonment issues of his own. He wanted the same things I did—to be loved and accepted. I saw myself in him so clearly. I had been lucky to have my mom to love and support me and protect me from his alcoholism.

I had two choices: either I could continue to blame him for my feelings, or I could empathize with a man who had struggled with addiction all his life. As a nurse in training, I consciously chose the latter.

Years later, when my dad was 55, he started attending AA meetings seriously. He finally had conquered the beast and was sober, and I finally met the man who was remorseful, loving and had God in his life. Four years later, at 59, he was diagnosed with cancer and died. He left me behind once again.

Changing Our Connection to Our Story

I have taken care of many alcoholic patients over the years. My heart goes out to them. Guess what else? They teach me about who my dad was through their story of struggle. I truly emphasize with them.

Once, a man named Chris came to see me. He was an alcoholic. His mother, Betty, was a patient too, as well as his wife, Teresa. Every time Chris came in, he talked about quitting drinking, believing he could do it on his own. I assured him that he could not and that he needed help. But he was in denial. He would get sober for a while and then return to drinking. Meanwhile, his wife was telling me her side of the story, which was quite different. When Betty came in, she would tell her side of the story. No one was on the same page. This went on for years, and I saw Chris' life fall apart. I felt so much compassion for him. His wife left him, he lost his job, and he moved in with his mother.

Then one visit, he told me he had reconnected with his high school sweetheart and he wanted help. I had told him the story of my dad many times, but this time, he heard that with AA, my dad got better and became a great guy. Chris wanted to be that great guy, and I was able to offer him hope.

This is why changing our connection to our story is so important. If I were still resentful toward my dad, I would have seen an alcoholic who was hopeless in Chris and have been unable to offer him help. Overcoming the emotional challenges with my father made me the empathetic health provider I am today.

Transcending our Stories

Storytelling is an ancient art form that has been used as a tool throughout time to express who we are and what we feel. Now that you've heard my story, you have a better understanding of who I am as a person. Perhaps you've begun to think of stories of your own that have made you feel the same way. Or maybe you've thought of things that you need to let go of, too.

As you just read, my story began with desertion, which led to intense anxiety and abandonment issues. Because I was able to change my story, I also was able to start a new life separate from the trauma of the past.

Everyone has stories; probably ones that cause pain every time they are relived. It is time to heal. It's going to be difficult, but in order to change that painful story, we need to amend it and do the forgiveness work. The way to do this is by finding the good lessons from stories, the silver linings.

Studies show that our stories are only 50% true. Which means that the other 50% we made up, whether it's the defensive mechanism of our own mind, or the lens in which we chose to see the story played out. Seeing your story as 50% true can help to alleviate the injustices. Seeing the truth can help each of us begin our journey toward healing, acceptance, and emotional freedom.

I personally became tired of my stories. I decided I am bigger than my story.

I am stronger than my past, my perceived experiences. I am a healer.

Our Patients' Stories

As nurses, we hear stories from our patients all day long. We hear about when the pain started, how immobilizing it is, and how they've tried to alleviate it.

A medical history is a story.

It's important to remember how scary it can be for our patients to come to the hospital or doctor's office. All they want is to be heard. Our job is to become an empathetic listener. By listening, we give the patient permission to tell their story in a safe place. It's good to remember there may be an underlying story.

Using Stories in Health Care

Health care centers are relying on the power of story more and more. There are endless ways in which hospitals are using stories to improve patient experiences, unite caregiver teams, and utilize data in new ways.

Northwell Health is a group of hospitals and outpatient centers in New York. The marketing team for this organization loves using a particular story to make an impact and grow its team.

The leader, Sven, received a comment from an unhappy patient about his organization. So he called the patient in for an interview. He also interviewed one of his happy customers. The contrast was apparent. He then combined the two interviews in a video and presented them to an entire room of the company's senior leaders. The team leaders were so moved that they continued to talk about the importance of stories for months.

If Only Stories

As we choose our life stories, keeping in mind that they may only be 50% accurate, we benefit from asking, what is missing? What is the other side of the story? What does our story say about us and our choices? Where do our stories leave us? Where do our stories lead us?

It is said that Dante Gabriel Rossetti, a famous 19th-century poet and artist, once was approached by a feeble, elderly man. The old fellow had brought some sketches and drawings that he wanted Rossetti to look at and tell him if they had any value, or if they at least showed potential talent.

Rossetti looked them over very carefully. After the first few, he knew they were worthless. They did not show any signs of artistic talent. But Rossetti was a kindhearted man, and he told the elderly man as gently as possible that the pictures were of no value. He was sorry, but he could not lie.

The visitor was disappointed, but he also seemed to expect Rossetti's judgment. He then apologized for taking up the great artist's time but wondered if he would look at a few other drawings that had been done by a much younger art student.

Rossetti analyzed the second batch of sketches and immediately became enthusiastic over the talent they revealed. "These," he said, "oh, these are excellent. This young student has real talent. He should be given every help and encouragement in his career to become an artist. He has a great future if he will just work hard and stick with it."

Rossetti could see that the old fellow was deeply touched.

"Do you know this fine young artist?" he asked. "Is it your son?" "No," said the old man sadly. "It is my work from over 40 years ago. If only I had heard such praise then! For you see, I got discouraged and gave up—much too soon."

This story is an example of how unfortunate it can be when our story is not told at the right time, listened to with openness, or encouraged. As nurses, we have perfect opportunities to elicit and listen to stories. A small word of encouragement from us may be just what is needed to change an 'if only' story into a positive life experience.

The Chemicals of Storytelling

Storytelling is packed full of emotional chemicals. Stories create empathy. And empathy creates oxytocin, better known as our feel-good chemical. Or, as I like to think of it, our emotional connector.

Paul Zak, a neuroeconomics expert, has done an outstanding job of researching empathy and connection: "As social creatures, we depend on others for our survival and happiness. My lab discovered that a neurochemical called oxytocin signals the brain that it's safe to approach others. Oxytocin is produced when we are trusted or shown a kindness, and it motivates cooperation with others. It does this by enhancing the sense of empathy, our ability to experience others' emotions."

When you and your patient tell each other stories, you will be chemically connected through the oxytocin in your brain. If you're able to find a story from your own life that has a happy ending, use it! You and the patient will enjoy a splash of happiness from the release of serotonin, dopamine, and oxytocin. Create your own story that stimulates their inner happy chemicals by starting out with pain and ending with promise. Stories reveal we are the solution to our problems.

David JP Phillips is another researcher who has delved into the chemical responses of storytelling. Phillips has identified that stories can affect both positive hormones and negative hormones, depending on what kind of story you tell. He describes the 'angel's cocktail' as serotonin, dopamine, and oxytocin. David explains that the 'devil's cocktail' has the hormones cortisol and adrenaline.

Oxytocin, which helps us become more generous, trust more and bond better, is created by stories that begin with struggle and end with meaningful solutions.

~

I use my medical story to help other people. I was 16 years old and in the hospital to have a mass in my breast the size of a grapefruit removed. I was scared I had cancer. My grandmother and my great-grandmother had both had breast cancer.

My mom left the hospital at 5 p.m.; shortly thereafter, I became violently sick to my stomach in fear and anticipation of my morning surgery. I was scared. I put my light on, and the nurse came in and told me I was NPO so I couldn't have anything by mouth. She also told me I didn't have any orders for pain medicine.

I called my mom and she tried to soothe me over the phone, but I wanted her to come back to the hospital. I felt alone. Misunderstood. I had nowhere to go. I was stuck in that hospital bed in those goofy pj's. I cried myself to sleep. I promised that I would never leave someone alone in the hospital and if someone needed me, I would show up. So, I tell patients this story:

I was in the hospital once and I was so afraid. I know how you feel. You may experience fear or pain while you are here. But in the end, you are going to be okay and you are going to go home happy and healthy. Then this will be just a memory. If you need me to help you with something, I won't let you down. I know when you're in the hospital you feel like no one is around because that's how I felt, but all you have to do is press this button and I will respond.

Now, they feel safe and trust me and together, we can control their pain and emotions. Connecting to each other through story releases stress for both of us. If the patients are calm, we are calm!

The Negative Chemicals

The negative chemicals adrenaline and cortisol come into play when stories are scary. Stories about cancer or surgery or even diabetes are scary. According to David Phillips, when we watch movies or hear stories that are negative, we may experience feelings of intolerance or irritability. Which is why I make it a habit to avoid violent or scary movies and stories. They get me wound up inside, and my heart begins to race.

Stories that are scary give us an adrenaline rush. I am reluctant to use negative stories to help patients try to get on track with their health. I used to tell them, "If you don't get these blood sugars down, you could lose your sight or toes." They would leave the office thinking, "These sugars are going to kill me." Not only that, but they walked out of the office having a very negative experience. The feeling of being scolded and 'not good enough' will not bring them back to the office any time soon. Now I remind them that it is in their power to manage their diabetes with diet and exercise, for example, and live a healthier life.

This positive story will bring them back.

The 7 Second Rule

We all want to feel connected and understood. As health care workers, we must make a great 7-second impression.[29] In 7 seconds, someone already has decided whether they like us or not. (By the way, you do the same.)

I've shared my first impression strategy using eye contact, the hand on the bottom handshake, touching a shoulder, matching the breathing of the client—all of this purposefully creates a positive connection. Try it! Learn it. Share it.

There is power in learning about our patients. When I meet someone new, I try to connect. I comment on something they are wearing that I like. I look at their face: do they have a nice smile, big eyes, or awesome hair?

When I see a male about my age, I ask about his kids. "Are they in college? Where?" Often, I will find a commonality: my kids are in college, too. I can talk about the cost, the lifestyle, the differences in having them out of the house. All of these connect us. If it is a female and she is a young mom, I can find one of my young mom stories. A flurry of activity taking them to school, sports, music, and how much fun or stress the hustle can be. I lived that story already.

Once I find the one thing we have in common, I am in and the conversation is smooth sailing. I have found and made my connections. Oxytocin begins to develop as vibrational energy connects me and the patient.

What is the Goal of Your Story?

When you are telling a story, always come up with the lesson you are trying to convey first. The lesson should be positive and encouraging for the other person.[30]

For example, if diabetes compliance is what you want to achieve with your patients, then you need to create the story that supports diabetes compliance.

I just happen to have a great diabetic story: When I was 10 years old, my best friend went to the hospital. I thought that hospitals were where you went to die. She was very sick with diabetes. I cried. I thought my best friend was going to die. In those days, you couldn't call or text people to see how they were. You relied on your parents to connect and then let you know.

After a few weeks in the hospital (yes, they did that back then), she came home and taught me about diabetes. She would eat tablespoons of butter or peanut butter depending on her blood sugar results. Not a meal, just a spoonful. I'm telling the truth here. Back in the 1970s, diabetics didn't live much past 20 years.

When I became a nurse practitioner, I began to use that story for my diabetic patients, told this way:

> *I once had a friend in grade school. She was 10 years old when she got diabetes. Can you **imagine** what that was like for her? I remember crying when I heard she was in the hospital. They kept her forever so I didn't think she would ever get better. Back then she wasn't expected to live past 20 years old, but she is still alive and is 57 now. The reason is **because** we have such great medications for diabetics today to keep blood sugars under control. I can help you learn to do that. **You** will become an excellent diabetic.*

Use Hypnotic Words in Your Story

Words are powerful indeed. Some words are hypnotic. They encourage an accepting frame of mind. In the above example, I bolded three words. These three words are words to include in your story to pack a punch.

Start with **imagine**. It's like seeing a dream or a future. Imagine you can do this. It is not a sales pitch, like "you must do this." It's more like "imagine if you controlled your diabetes and you didn't get neuropathy."

You is the person's name card. When you use the word "you" it reinforces that the topic of conversation—the story—is only about that one person. Everyone likes to hear their name, and "you" is the same as saying the person's name and is less intrusive. Once I had a patient who used my name in every other sentence. It drove me crazy. It's better to use the word "you" and then periodically use their name. Overusing a stranger's name makes them uncomfortable.

Because is a word that has cause and effect. When you use "because," you are satisfying the brain's natural appeal for reasons.

Why Use Your Own Story?

Ask yourself this question: "Can I create a story that is so personal that it can help people change?" If you answer yes, do the following (see graphic below):

1. Take out a piece of paper and draw a line across the paper from left to right.
2. Label the left 'birth' and label the right 'today.'
3. Tick off 10-year increments on the paper to represent your life span.
4. On that grid, write out milestones that have occurred in your life.
5. Analyze what you have learned from the lessons contained in your life events—your story.
6. For each event, write out what lesson you have learned from that event.
7. There will be many to choose from. If you have tragic events and you feel uncomfortable with this process, skip them. Do not just replay a tragic event.

The Lifeline

If I want to tell a story to my patients who are dealing with stress from a difficult childhood, I look at my timeline.

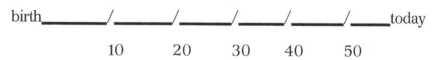

The goal is to share a story that can help another person learn a better way of seeing and doing something. Now, identify the stories you have been telling.

- Are they positive or negative?
- Do you want to look at them and see them another way?

- Are they your best stories?

By the time I was 10, I had overdosed on aspirin, had my stomach pumped, had over 20 stitches in my leg, and my dad had moved.

By the time I was 20, I had been in a robbery twice, had breast surgery…you get the idea.

Now use your stories to create a 30-second pitch oozing with positivity that will help someone.

The Hero's Journey

The Hero's Journey appeals to people because it reminds them of their higher potential. In his 1949 book, *The Hero With a Thousand Faces*, cultural anthropologist Joseph Campbell argues that the world's great myths and creation stories follow the same basic plot:

- Life in the village is normal until one day an urgent problem arises, such as a menacing dragon.
- A hero accepts the challenge and goes on a quest to find and slay the dragon.
- Obstacles arise along the way, and the hero considers giving up.
- But in a moment of insight, the hero realizes what must be done to succeed.
- Our hero musters the resolve to slay the dragon and returns home triumphant, with new knowledge and experience.
- Order is restored.

StoryBrand[31] is a marketing firm that helps create stories for a business or product. Here is the StoryBrand framework for you to try to create your story:

- A patient/hero
- Has a problem

- And meets a guide
- Who has a plan
- That calls them to action
- That helps them avoid failure
- And ends up with success.

Create (or Recreate) Your Story

Think about your life and the stories you have told and retold. Do any of your stories need to be repaired? Restructured? Reformed?

Write out your timeline and look at the various events in your life. Use the timeline stories to look for lessons. Anything on your timeline can be changed to reflect something better. Remember, whatever story you tell reinforces how the brain perceives those events: good or bad.

Write down your new stories. Think about when you might use them and with which patients.

Enlist stories from your patients. Ask yourself how their story makes you feel.

Start telling your story using The Hero's Journey. Give them *HOPE: Heart, Optimism, Pause, and Energy* to be well.

Chapter Twelve

The Power of Peers (SMAs)

Find a group of people who challenge and inspire you,
spend a lot of time with them, and it will change your life.
— Amy Poehler

Until now, this book has explored many powerful types of tools and techniques to help our patients. I am not immune to the time war that is going on in our industry. As we discussed earlier, we are doing more charting and less one-on-one care. I began to search for another way to help me stay true to my mission to help educate and eradicate disease. I too have to be conscientious about how much time I spend with patients, but I refuse to allow the clock to keep me from teaching my patients breath work, meditation procedures, and self-care energy work.

What could possibly be the solution?

How are we doing as a medical profession?

Health care is changing quickly. We are no longer allowed to linger in the room with a patient. We have criteria that we have to document and more visits that have to be done.

The Dilemma

I check Catherine's chart; she is new to our practice, and she is 60 years old.

"Good morning, Catherine!" I stretch out my hand, connect with my eyes (silently, "I love you.") and ask her to have a seat in the chair as I touch her on the shoulder lightly. She is a well-dressed woman with a beautiful smile. "How can I help you today?"

She tells me she hasn't seen a provider in a long time. She has been very thirsty and has to go to the bathroom constantly. She thinks she has a urine infection.

She admits that she ran out of blood pressure medication sometime last year.

She doesn't check her blood pressure because she feels fine.

I check her blood sugar, and it calculates in at 292, her blood pressure 170/96. The red light goes off in my head like a siren. I quickly begin to formulate a plan of care. I complete her new patient packet and begin her physical exam. I hear the timer go off in the hallway, alerting me that my time is up. I breathe and think to myself, what a mess. Running against the timer, I try to discuss her diagnosis with her when tears begin to run down her cheek. She tells me her mother had diabetes and lost her leg.

She looks me square in the eye and asks me, "Am I going to lose my leg?"

I shake my head no. I hold her hand, I softly tell her she is going to be okay, and she is not going to lose her leg. We need to concentrate on getting the blood sugar and blood pressure numbers down. I try to console her and at the same time, I know I have to finish up.

The problems Catherine faces are numerous. She needs to check her blood sugars at home. She doesn't even know what a glucometer is or where to get one.

Her blood pressure is elevated, so she needs to use a blood pressure monitor so she can check that at home, too. She needs new medications and an explanation of what they are, when to take them, and what the side effects might be.

We are both overwhelmed. How do I empower her to take the lead in reducing her risk factors from diabetes, hypertension, and obesity? It would take me 10 visits to feed her the information she needs to travel the road of wellness. I feel stressed as I walk out of the room and realize that there are three patients waiting to be seen. I shake my head, knowing now I have to play catch up and apologize to patients who also deserve their time, too.

~

Eighteen years have passed since I became a nurse practitioner. I have never felt so rushed and so overwhelmed with patients' numerous health issues, and so inefficient in helping patients get control of their health problems.

Providers have to increase the number of patients seen in a day just to keep their practices alive financially. I see patients getting sicker, with fewer resources, higher copays, and very little knowledge about the science of health.

Because they can't afford to come in, they let their medications run out. They don't feel bad, so they assume they are fine. They stop checking their blood sugars because it hurts to prick their finger, but little do they know, they are slowly killing themselves.

I had to find a solution—not just for my stress level, but for all of my patients who deserve to live long and healthy lives but can't without good education, lifestyle interventions, and time to discuss their issues.

I had heard about Shared Medical Appointments (SMAs) from my vitamin sales rep, Kristen. She had been harping on me for years to start group visits at my practice. I had to do something to help patients learn that they can make different decisions about their health. I wanted to help them implement changes to combat the devastating effects of diseases.

I also wanted to help myself. I wanted to be able to provide the kind of health care I thought patients deserved and needed. After researching SMAs, I decided to take the leap and start them at my practice.

Shared Medical Appointments (SMAs)

SMAs are scheduled sessions or appointments that include a group of patients that 1) you care for on a regular basis, and 2) share the same health concerns, e.g., diabetes, stress and anxiety, pain, smoking, etc.

Think about it. If you work in a nephrology clinic, you can schedule your patient for a group visit to teach them all about different types of dialysis. If you have a renal patient who is not ready for dialysis but needs to be on a renal diet and receive renal vitamins, that would be a different group. The provider, the nurse, or the medical assistant can help run the sessions. The main criteria is that the practitioner is present to assess the patients and provide a billable service, which includes a subjective, objective assessment and plan (SOAP), just like your one-on-one appointments.

SOAP Notes

Consider an SMA with a diabetic group. First, we give them a handout with the diabetic assessment questions. This meets the 'subjective' findings and includes the date of their last eye exam and foot exam. We ask questions about neuropathy, current blood sugar numbers taken at home, and how often they check. We get their vital signs, blood sugar and A1C. If due, we will obtain their yearly urine microalbumin specimen. This helps us meet the 'objective findings.' Then we begin the SMAs by focusing on what patients need to do to improve their blood glucose levels. I also use this 60- to 90-minute visit to give them demonstrations of what they should be doing with their diet. I show them bags of sugar that represent the foods we most commonly eat and drink. We read labels, discuss blood sugar goals, and learn about hemoglobin A1C's. We troubleshoot glucometer testing. I also facilitate time for patients to educate each other while I do mini exams, look over their questionnaires, and address concerns. The 'assessment and plan' are completed after I look at all of their vital signs, blood sugar levels, and meds. This concludes the necessary documentation for a visit.

Shared medical appointments became a solution for my practice when I wanted to give more time than I was allotted. Because of cuts in reimbursements by insurance, we are unable to adequately address all of a patient's concerns in a single one-on-one appointment. Shared medical appointments offer patients more time to focus on a strategy to initiate self-care changes. They bring together patients with common disease processes and introduce lifestyle interventions to help patients make better and healthier choices. I love facilitating dialogue between patients to discuss their health concerns.

An amazing thing I see happen in these visits are patients connecting with each other. At the end of the last SMA, one of the members asked if anyone wanted to start a group text message. Everyone was interested, so she took their numbers and started a patient discussion group. They began walking together at the local college. I was thrilled to see how the SMAs created camaraderie. It was so awesome to watch people helping and healing together. This was a feel-good moment.

How to Implement a Billable SMA

The best way to implement a successful, billable SMA is to check out Lifestyle Matrix at lifestylematrix.com. Here, you can purchase pre-made group visit forms and videos along with billable notes. They sell kits that give you directions for the SMA visits.

I merged my practice, and the new owners were very hesitant about group visits. I have been doing SMAs for years, so I had no reservations whatsoever. But to help them become comfortable, I put together all of the data and presented them with the scientific research.

Then I called Lifestyle Matrix to set up an appointment with one of their representatives and my managers. I also copied the 99213 criteria and prepared the note to reflect the criteria we must meet.

So do your homework and learn about SMAs, implement them, and become the patient advocate at your office or place of employment. Don't back down if you believe they would help your patients. Nothing is ever going to change unless we change. We have to take the lead and demand a new health care approach for our patients and ourselves.

Another option would be to purchase the book, *Running Group Visits in Your Practice* by Edward B. Noffsinger that gives you the outline and permission to institute group visits in your practice.

In the words of Mahatma Gandhi, "Be the change you wish to see in the world." That means stand up to the status quo and demand something different to help patients heal. I have hope that all of us will do our part to spread the emerging community of SMAs that is so desperately needed.

Documentations and Billing

Documentation is the key (as it is with all billable charges). We typically bill a 99213, but if that bothers you, do a 99212. I know some providers bill a 99214.

There is not a clear delineation of the SMA criteria, which I think is why people shy away from doing them. But let's not be scared! Let's get educated and begin helping our patients and our communities.

The 99213 code is considered an Evaluation and Management of an established patient when the provider of service meets two of the following three criteria: expanded problem; focused history, expanded problem; focused exam, low medical decision making.

Diabetes group visits are presented as an expanded problem with a focused history and exam, the medical decision-making is low, the presenting problem is low to moderate severity. If you still are not sure about the billing, simply go online and make sure your office notes for this visit meets the criteria at cgsmedicare.com/partb/mr/pdf/99213.pdf.

Who Is Doing SMAs?

According to the American Academy of Family Physicians, only 12.7% of family physicians conducted group visits in 2010. While it was up from 7% in 2005, we could be doing so much better. There is a need that we can fill.

Why We Need Better Solutions

Let's look at one disease state to see the impact SMAs could have on the health care system and the patients.

- In 2017, the total estimated cost of diagnosed diabetes in the U.S. was $327 billion.

- In 2016, a total of 16 million emergency department visits were reported with diabetes as one of the listed diagnoses among adults aged 18 years or older.

- Someone is diagnosed with diabetes every 2 minutes. *Yikes.*

- 88 million American adults—approximately 1 in 3—have prediabetes.

- According to a study in 2010, diabetes cuts off an average 8.5 years from the lifespan of a 50-year-old man compared to one without. This doesn't even account for the blindness, dialysis, neuropathy, stroke, paralysis, etc.

The CDC and Diabetic Group Visits

The CDC supports diabetic lifestyle change programs like SMAs and group visits because research shows that's what works. They did a randomized clinical study that showed those who completed the lifestyle change program reduced their chances of developing type 2 diabetes by 58% compared to the placebo group (71% for individuals 60 and older). That's nearly twice as much as the reduction among the group taking metformin (31%). A follow-up study showed that participants were still one-third less likely to develop type 2 diabetes a decade later than individuals who took a placebo. Those who did develop type 2 diabetes delayed the onset of the disease by about four years. Pretty impressive.

Providers Learn, Too

One of the things I learned from group visits is that people drink 2 liters of soda a day. I learned they like Twinkies and cupcakes for breakfast along with coffee with sugar and cream. A whole bag of chips is devoured in one sitting, and no one knows that is not a serving size. I learned that it's not one piece of chicken, but three or four pieces at a meal. I learned that people go home after work and relax in bed with a refrigerator filled with goodies next to them instead of a nightstand. They thought this was a creative solution for going to the kitchen for a snack since they spend most of their time in bed.

I was shocked. Until I started group meetings, I had no idea what was causing all of the diabetes, hypertension, and obesity. Learning from the patients about what they are commonly doing wrong allows me to demystify the current advertising gimmicks of the food industry. I love discussing the food industry's marketing plans to sabotage our health. I remind patients that the food industry is in it to make money, and they provide what we crave.

My first year doing SMAs I lectured at patients for an hour before I learned to be more of a facilitator. Now I have the Conversation Map Tools.[32] I hand out cards with questions on them and allow each patient to take turns reading them. Then, I allow the group to problem solve. It is impressive to hear the patients offer each other advice. They really want to help each other.

Stress Group Visits

When I first started doing group visits, a lot of things complicated the process. One day I was eavesdropping on the receptionist's conversation. The receptionist, Jenny, was explaining to the patient that anyone on controlled medication for anxiety must attend a group visit. Pause. "That is our office policy." Pause. "If you want your refill, you will have to attend the group visit." Long pause, then Jenny hangs up.

I ask her, "What was that all about?"

Jenny was very aggravated from being yelled at on the phone. "Laurie said you can't hold her Xanax hostage!" Instead of giving in, we stick with our policy. Fast forward to the day of the group visit on stress and self-help. Laurie sits in the corner with a frown on her face, her arms are crossed, and she is not interested in conversing with anyone. She just wants her prescription. The group meeting begins, and I start with how the fight and flight process causes stress on the body. We discuss the symptoms of a panic attack and how that relates to the chemicals and hormones in our body. I also discuss the learned stress responses. I saw her ears perk up.

We went through coping strategies. I gave a demonstration of physical strategies to move the lymphatics, the hormones, and the vagus nerve and had each patient create a power pose. I facilitated relaxation through heart breathing exercises and a short meditation intertwined with my hypnosis scripts. I also provided patients with handouts for vitamin options, oils to diffuse, and sleep strategies. The meeting ends, and I write scripts and do my charting.

The following morning, Laurie calls Jenny to say she is so sorry for how she acted about coming to the group meeting. She complimented the whole process and ended with, "I called my sister and told her she needed to do the group visit, too!"

Her heart won over by SMAs, she will become our billboard. As an office, we were able to enjoy another "well done" compliment.

We made a ripple, we made a difference.

The group visits are so powerful. They help patients learn how to calm themselves in the midst of chaos. For me, they are always about what I can give the patients to help them be a better and healthier version of themselves. It's about individualizing the SMAs to address our patients' needs.

I like to think of them as Brain Empowerment visits. Anyone can benefit from a group stress meeting, especially since studies show that 80% to 90% of patients' complaints have some kind of emotional component to them. One out of 4 people are on antidepressants.

In my practice, once patients are put on medication for depression, they rarely come off. That's why upfront education is imperative to understand the choices and perhaps prevent a lifetime of antidepressant use. Patients also refuse to go to counseling, and no one wants to see a psychiatrist. That is where we come in as nurses and providers. We can set a policy on how to implement SMAs, then stand by the policy. We encourage and influence them to participate in the group visits. This is where the real juice of healing is going to happen. This may be the only time the patients are going to hear what is causing their symptoms, how to control them, and begin to advocate for their own health. Instead of being victimized by the food industry or stress, we help them understand meditation, hypnosis, art, movement, dance, prayer, depression scales, mini mental exams, and other holistic care in our group visits.

Community

Community gets the blue ribbon when it comes to increasing longevity.

When researchers looked at key components for longevity, community was ranked at the top, which makes SMAs an even greater tool for our patients. In the community setting, people connect, communicate, and share with each other. This can be especially important as we age, since older adults may have fewer connections and loneliness can set in.

Facilitating the group sessions is also an excellent way to build provider skills, increase awareness, and better engage with patients. I like to assign tasks to the members of the group as another way to get them involved. This helps them remember the information presented. I'll have one person be the timer, another the secretary, and another in charge of handing out the literature. I also start with an icebreaker to make people comfortable and start conversations. I want to make these as fun and enjoyable as I can. I want patients to feel good, to come be part of a group with the intention of healing.

How Much Can a Patient Absorb in One Visit?

This is an important question. When patients enter our office or the hospital, they are already set up for failure. They are nervous, they have very little knowledge about medicine, and their attention span is minimal. Studies show that patients' actual recall of information they obtained from our visits with them are startlingly low: approximately 40% to 80% of the medical information we give patients is forgotten immediately. The greater the amount of information, the lower the proportion that is correctly recalled. Furthermore, what they do remember is 50% incorrect.[33]

This data reinforces the need for a more casual environment that utilizes group education to help patients better comprehend some of the more complex issues involved in disease management. During SMAs the provider can encourage patients to write things down, which is a great memory reinforcement technique. The use of pictography, pictures with actions, is also a great learning tool. I encourage patients to repeat back to me the major learning highlights at the end.

And I use neuro-linguistic programming (NLP) as presented in Chapter Four. NLP elicits ideas and stimulates thought processes among the patients as they discuss wellness and health strategies. The motivational interviewing questions can be used to help patients identify and resolve issues.

I have seen firsthand how one-on-one appointments become repetitious because providers are not always able to build from one visit to the next, sometimes because the patient is non-compliant, or they haven't kept up with their visits. Typically, I see no improvement in blood pressure or in blood sugar levels. The reasons are numerous, but at the end of the day, I think it is a lack of understanding what is really going on with their bodies. They don't feel awful, so they are not motivated to invest in making big lifestyle changes.

Most patients have limited information about their health and need healthy behavior interventions. Newer research suggests that genetics are not actually what causes most of our health issues. Some research says lifestyle is the cause of disease 79% of the time, and other research states it may be as high at 95%. If our genetics are only responsible for diseases 5% to 30% of the time, it makes a lot of sense to start positioning lifestyle education into all disease-driven SMAs.

Which brings me back to SMAs and a study that looked at chronically ill patients. The patients that were in the SMAs cost the health care system $41.80 less and had higher satisfaction scores, fewer hospital admissions and better quality of life. This adds up to a lot of positives and a lot of dollars.

I think it's exciting that SMAs make our practice different. We are supporting our patients, adding value to their lives, and having a trickle-down effect for a healthier community.

My interest in group visits was reinforced when a patient stopped me after the session and thanked me for everything I do for her as a provider. She went on to say, "You go above and beyond to help your patients. This meeting was great, and you really contribute a lot of your time to us. We appreciate it."

I thanked her and told her I am not special and that I get paid for my time to do group visits.

"Yes," she said, "but no one else is doing them. You really care."

Now doesn't that sound like a good way to promote a practice and heal patients?

So, it's time to figure out how to create one in your health care setting. They can be used for anything: pain management, pre-surgery instructions, pre-dialysis unit introduction, laboratory review for diabetes, cholesterols, thyroid, Genova labs, Medicare Wellness, pro-time clinic guidelines—the value of the group formation is endless.

When scientists began tracking the health of 268 Harvard sophomores in 1938 during the Great Depression, they hoped the longitudinal study would reveal clues to how to be happy and successful. After following the surviving 'Crimson Men' for nearly 80 years, the one thing that stood out the most was relationships. That's it. Not money, not where you live or how prestigious your job was, but how successful you were in relationships. Simple, right? We arrive right back at the community of groups and relationships.

Loneliness

Steve Cole, Ph.D., director of the Social Genomics Core Laboratory at the University of California-Los Angeles, offers up the physiology of loneliness. He explains that "loneliness acts as a fertilizer for other diseases. The biology of loneliness can accelerate the buildup of plaque in arteries, help cancer cells grow and spread, and promote inflammation in the brain leading to Alzheimer's disease. Loneliness promotes wear and tear on the body. Some researchers believe loneliness can reduce a life span by eight years, revealing that social isolation creates a heavy disease burden. Enter a group and relate with others.

What the Studies Show

Kaiser Permanente conducted a one-year pilot study on Drop-In Group Medical Appointments (DIGMAs) in the Colorado region. They found that 90% of the patients who attended reported being satisfied with the DIGMA visits and more than 60% of patients stated that they would **not** have preferred an individual office visit.

Cleveland Clinic's provided 10 weeks of group visits. They showed that patients had improved health outcomes, and 85% of patients attending a DIGMA rescheduled their next appointment to another DIGMA visit. The patients rated their overall satisfaction with their visit as much higher for DIGMA, with 74.6% preferring DIGMAs over individual office visits with the same provider (59.1%).

Lifestyle Medicine Movement!

SMAs bring people together to create a sense of community, a community of patients that can work together to increase disease prevention and explore healthy living options. Some SMAs literally bring in other community health leaders to educate and promote healthy lifestyles. There is great power in groups.

In a medical practice, the practitioner can identify patients who have poor support systems and connect them with a group where they may get motivated, feel welcomed by others, and in the process, reduce the side effects of diseases and loneliness. The benefits are numerous:

- You can overbook to accommodate no call/no shows. Expect about 50% no shows in the beginning.
- They are relaxed and informative; you set the tone and style.
- They reduce the burden of disease.
- You get to know your patients better.
- They are fun for patients and providers.

- They have a ripple effect by spreading information to patients who then spread information to families and communities.
- You can implement stress reduction processes.
- They have higher levels of satisfaction.
- They assist in generating revenue.
- They help establish you as a provider who sees that health care is a commitment and that you are here to help patients get better. Patients see you as valuable and spread the word.
- They provide a type of group therapy.
- You can be as creative as you would like to be.
- You spend more time addressing the real burden of disease.
- You save money for insurance and the government.
- More intimate conversation happens regarding illness and wellness.
- They allow providers time to educate patients and find outpatients' real concerns.
- They create greater patient compliance with medical management.
- They reduce the number of outpatient specialty and emergency room visits.
- They reduce the number of hospital admissions.
- Providers and patients have higher satisfaction scores.
- You can implement stress reduction techniques, pain reduction techniques, diabetes reduction techniques, etc.

- You can impact unhealthy communities by educating patients and asking them to help someone else. A pass it forward approach.

- They place your practice in the elite group of ones that really impact health.

- You can collaborate with other providers and specialties to incorporate their services into the shared medical appointments. This could include dance, nutritionist, shopping list, therapist, nurse, and health coach. The ideas are limitless.

- They combat isolation.

- Patients feel inspired by other people's stories and journeys of illness and wellness.

- You provide cutting-edge care for your patients.

Note: Shared Medical Appointments (SMAs) offer a valuable approach to engaging patients in group sessions so they can get more disease-based information while sharing their experiences. While the SMAs can be held in a virtual setting to accommodate pandemic protocols, keep in mind that this was written for implementation pre-pandemic and is therefore not as immediately applicable. Also consider that it takes three months to get group visits up and running. It may be that by the time you write the protocols and recruit the patients, the pandemic may be over. Hold your hat; don't give up yet. This would be the perfect time to gather information and establish ideas.

See the appendix to find free resources and learn how to implement your own shared medical appointments.

Chapter Thirteen

The Gift

Let us realize that: the privilege to work is a gift,
the power to work is a blessing, the love of work is success!
–David O. McKay

My calling is to serve people everywhere by providing hope and the light of God to reveal that he shines in all of us. All we have to do is show up, learn one, and teach one.

I hope you think about doing that, too. If you are young, you have a whole life of family and fun ahead of you. If you are older, you understand that now can be your comeback to greatness. Add some new techniques to energize what you do and who you are. No one expects you to do them all, but do purposefully have fun, always trying to be better and unique.

I want to encourage you to keep working at your craft, whatever it may be. Search for your God-given purpose and be compelled by your heart, be encouraged that you can develop the potential that is undoubtedly within you.

Look for someone you can encourage. That someone will look back in the years to come with gratitude to the kindness and generous care that propelled them to their greatness. I love the following story:

Once upon a time, a young girl was walking through a
meadow and saw a beautiful butterfly impaled on a thorn.
Very carefully and lovingly she released the butterfly until it
was able to fly away. But then it came back and magically

changed into a fairy princess. "Because you were so kind to me," said the fairy princess to the small girl, "I will grant you one wish." The little girl thought, and then replied, "I want to be happy all the time!" The fairy princess leaned in toward her and whispered in her ear, and then she vanished. As the girl began to grow older, she became happier and happier. No one else in the land was nearly as happy. Whenever anyone asked what her secret to happiness was, she would only smile and say, "I listened to a good fairy princess." As she reached the last years of her life, her friends became afraid that her fabulous secret for happiness might die with her. "Tell us, tell us please!" they begged her. "Tell us your secret to happiness. Tell us what the good fairy princess said." The lovely older lady smiled warmly, and then she replied, "The good fairy princess whispered into my ear these words, 'Everyone has need of you, no matter how secure they may seem. Everyone has need of you, please answer the calling.'" (Revised from the book, The One Year Love Talk Devotional for Couples)

This is true for us, too. Everyone has a need for us. That little girl believed it, nurtured it, ingrained it and became it. She focused so much on those precious words. It was in the practice over and over again. "Everyone has a need for me, no matter what." I try to always answer the calling. Will you?

Sometimes we don't see the changes right away, but in a year, if you practice even one thing you learned, you will be able to look back and see the truth of it all. You are the light, you are the truth, you are the way. Go ahead! Start just one thing today. Be a healer.

Chapter Fourteen

Weaving It All Together

*Sometimes when we think it's the end of the road
is when we learn to fly.*
—Mimi Novic, *Guidebook to Your Heart*

Practice does not make perfect, it makes permanent.
—Vince Lombardi

Writing this book has been a uniquely challenging endeavor. I've opened myself up, sharing and describing my own and others' stories. I have written about crying when I listened to Leo Buscaglia talk about love at a time when I was feeling so alone after being cheated on and dumped. And how, in a state of sadness, I pondered what Dr. Wayne Dyer was teaching me about love and creating positive intentions. I used all of the teachings of Tony Robbins and Dr. Joe Dispenza to try to control my whacked-out thoughts and ideas about the world.

I wrote about my own lost hope and asked myself what more I could do. In asking, I discovered the threads of my story were too negative for me to ever build a beautiful future. That's when the heavy lifting really began.

I worked to correct my thoughts through self-hypnosis. I wrote new thought scripts. I felt raw energy building inside of me for the first time, and that put me on the path of healing my chakras and meridians.

I wanted better relationships at home and at work. Learning NLP and MI corrected many of my relationship issues by removing communication barriers and creating real connections.

I wanted to feel closer to God, and *A Course in Miracles* landed on my bookshelf.

I searched for others who could help me, and I found wonderful coaches: Gina Nicole, Kristen Brokaw, Barbara Goodman Siegel, Stacey O'Byrne, Dawn Ferguson, Cheryl Oliver, Stacy Fidler, Tom Hill, Cathy Davis and so many more. Every teacher imprinted my life in some way, and now, a part of them exists in me. My family—Ken, Sadie, Jaime and David— have also taught me valuable lessons about who I am and who I want to become. They are the basis of my existence, and I constantly learn lessons from them that are so valuable to me. They fill my heart with a love so great that I have to share it with the world. And it's worked that way with patients as well. Many of my patients have taught me how to be a better mother and wife. They all have changed me and now I want to change you, too.

I am amazed at the cycles of life and opportunities for learning. All the things I have learned show up somewhere, sometime. I reflect over the stages of my life like the chapters of this book. I know that each skill I learned as a person, a wife, a mother, and a nurse was a chapter of my life. Each idea showed me the way to the next great gift.

I know that I want to be the best health group facilitator on the planet. I could not be that in Chapter One when I didn't even know how to love myself, let alone other people. I sure couldn't be that if I did not appreciate the pause of meditation that takes me to solitude, prayer, and patience. Certainly, listening and having empathy allows me to expand the learning in group settings.

Prior to my life of self-awareness, I was a mess. I moved from one thing to another, I was anxious and unsure of who I was. Basically, my energy could not be contained or focused. I ran, I jumped, I moved,

I danced. Finally, I learned that slowing down is necessary in order to hear, feel, see, and just be present. I learned to be silent so I could hear my spirit, recognize my calling, and understand my family and patients. I became attuned to my pains and my rhythms, which are often the pains and rhythms others experience.

I changed because other healers and leaders, writers and teachers stepped up their game and started a revolution among their own kind. I read about it, watched it, and incorporated it into my life.

As I finish this book, my 18-year career as a nurse practitioner at Chambers Medical Group has come to an end. It was a job I totally loved, and I miss it every day. The shift from a job that I loved to nothingness was startling. It left a huge gaping hole in my life. It also left time for me to assess my life and change, yet again.

The work I am doing now through consulting, teaching, writing, blogging, and working with patients uses everything I've learned. Writing this book has helped bring it all together. It can be summed up as asking questions, searching for answers. As I finish writing this book, I envision my life without the world I knew so well and loved so passionately for 18 years. While I feel sadness, it is clear to me that this ending is a beginning. I am so full of love for my patients and their families. I cherish their stories. We are missing each other. Therefore, I am sending out a gift of love and prayer to them right here and right now, so I can grieve and begin to move on. I send gratitude for all the lessons they taught me about how to be a better version of myself as a human, a nurse, a provider, and teacher.

As I let go of the family I made in medicine, I recognize that I have accepted many new truths and patched my heart, as well as others', through the years. That's what nurses do. They patch the hearts of other people with their own. I also am grateful that patients patch our hearts, too!

We affect many people, including generations to come. Mark Merrill writes, "How a parent raises their child—the love they give, the values they teach, the emotional environment they offer, the education they provide—influences not only their children, but the four generations to follow." I believe nurses and providers do the same thing. We influence generations to come. Everything we do matters; and remember, doing nothing is an action, too.

You Are One in a Billion

The probability of any of us being here is one in a billion. How is that possible?

In a single ejaculation, a man produces between 40 million and 1.2 billion sperm cells. That means each of us fought a war to get here. We were missioned to this earth with a purpose and a passion to make a difference.

Why do I mention this? Because we forget that each of us is unique. We all have the ability to spread love and understanding in the world like no one else. Everything we choose in our lives is up to us. Every encounter, every interaction has meaning and purpose; something is left behind, good or bad.

I'm inviting you to stay present and use this book as a manual to help you become the best version of yourself, to pamper yourself, heal yourself, and then take that light out into the world and become the best and healthiest version of yourself so you can lead others home, too. Set yourself up by applying these principles one at a time, practicing and staying true to who you are. Be amazing, be the blessing you want to see in others. Live with no regrets, and always wonder what amazing adventure is right around the corner. If you heal, another will see what you do and want to be like you! Congratulations, healers, on who you are and who you are becoming. I love you!

APPENDIX A

Daily Work Rituals

Here is an example of my daily work rituals. This may help you put it all together.

1. I open my eyes and say thank you to God for another day to play. I put my hands over my heart, then breathe in love and breathe out love.
2. I drink a full glass of water.
3. I am off to meditate at 5:30 a.m. for an hour in my closet. I do different types of meditation depending on what I am working on. Right now, I am doing the healing code for 15 minutes, reading a verse of ACIM, writing out my card, and doing work with Dr. Joe Dispenza.
4. I go outside and run for an hour. While I run, I go through Tony's 3 things: 3 minutes of gratitude, 3 minutes of thankful prayers, 3 minutes of how my day will be amazing. I am done by 7:30.
5. I take all of my vitamins consisting of turmeric, DIM, mitocore, glucosamine, fish oil, and vitamins B and D.
6. I make a smoothie with kale, spinach, broccoli, banana, blueberries, chia seeds, cinnamon, cayenne pepper, and almond milk.
7. I go to work and fill up my diffuser with essential oils. I apply the essential oils to my skin so I can breathe them in throughout the day.

8. Before I enter each patient's room, I stop, breathe, and focus.

9. I walk in, look them in the eyes with *I love you,* and shake their hand.

10. We sit on an equal level to develop rapport.

11. I apply some MI questions while watching their NLP language.

12. I use my NLP techniques to communicate.

13. I do my exam, allowing my hand to hover over any areas that are causing pain; if they don't have any, I hover my hand over one of their chakras. If I am doing an abdominal exam, I hover my hand over their solar plexus.

14. I discuss the care plan, and if time allows, I will teach them one tool, usually meditation, tapping, or diet, or I will refer them to a group visit so they can learn multiple things.

15. Throughout the day, I remind myself I am love. I use lunch to practice breathing or I do that on my bathroom breaks. I have been known to lay down and meditate during lunch time, too.

16. As I end my day, I use the same eye contact, warm touch and motivational NLP questions with my family.

17. I take my nighttime vitamins: probiotic, liver support, melatonin.

18. As I shut my eyes, I remember what I am grateful for that happened during my day. I then ask that my dreams be filled with answers to guide me to my soul purpose.

APPENDIX B

Power Tools for Nurses

I've referenced a variety of health modalities in this book. The following are additional resources to help in your learning to enhance your own and others' healing.

I also invite you to visit my website, donnanaumann.com, to contact me for additional support.

Biofeedback: Biofeedback is a system that helps take you from a place of stress to a place of balance and restoration. It is a form of monitoring your physiology. First monitor your physiology, then add in a relaxation technique, and then re-monitor your physiology. The FDA has approved RESPeRATE to help lower blood pressures. It is a breathing app with a belt and headphones that you wear to help synchronize your breathing and slow it down, which causes a reduction in blood pressure. The HeartMath app is another great biofeedback system that includes breathing techniques.

Gratitude: Gratitude is the biggest contributor to happiness. There are approximately 420,000 study results on Google Scholars exploring the benefits of gratitude and happiness.

Heart Breathing Exercise: Find a quiet place to sit and practice this technique.

1. Take a few deep breaths and relax. Focus your breathing by inhaling to the count of five, holding for five, blowing out to the count of five and, again, holding for five counts. Repeat.

2. Focus on your heart, and imagine your breath going in and coming out of your heart.

3. Continue this heart breathing.

4. Visualize someone you love or admire.

5. Place a picture of this person in your heart.

6. With this picture, continue focusing on your heart and breathing.

7. Feel what it is like to love, respect, and care for this person.

8. Place those feelings in your heart with the picture and continue breathing.

9. Now send that person the feelings you have in your heart. With each exhale, see this positive, loving energy going out to that person from all the cells of your body, from your heart.

10. On the inhale receive loving energy from the person you love. Receiving love is as important as giving love.

11. Continue with this exercise as long as you feel a positive response from your heart.

Heart Chakra Meditation, Essential Oils and Breath Work: Our heart chakra is the energy center that supports us. It sits in the middle of our chest. This chakra radiates love and connects the lower and higher chakras. It is a connection of the higher self and the earthly matters.

1. Use meditation to open your heart chakra. As you meditate, imagine spinning the energy wheel of the heart chakra clockwise, down the left and up the right. Relax into the feeling.

2. Apply essential oils or put them in a diffuser to amplify the meditation effects.

3. Put a drop of oil in your hands and breath in through your nose slowly, relaxing into the fragrance.

4. Add a mantra to your breath work. Something like "I am love," "I am loved," "I love and accept myself," or "Love surrounds me in all circumstances."

5. Place your hands over your heart in the center of your chest, close your eyes, and visualize the color green, repeating the mantra "love, peace, joy." Envision energy flowing up from your feet toward your heart and out through the top of your head. Run the energy down your arms and send it back to your heart through your palms as they lay on your heart.

Love Vibration: Dr. Shirley Marshall, Ph.D., author of the book Sacred Secrets writes:

"When we live in the love vibration, our energy resonates at a high frequency and we express the God qualities of compassion, forgiveness, tolerance, respect, generosity, joy, peace—all that inspires, empowers and enhances life. The love vibration lifts us to a higher state of consciousness and frees us of the thoughts, feelings, and actions that minimize and victimize us. Gone are any neurotic fear, guilt, judgment, greed, envy, arrogance, and the ego's stubborn need to be right. "Vexations of the spirit" lose their power over us. Free from the baggage of negativity and limited thinking, we begin to feel lighter and shine brighter. We become the magnet attracting our good."

Learn One, Teach One

- Sign up with HeartMath and challenge your team or department to teach themselves first, then the patients. HeartMath can calm someone before a procedure or surgery. It can help with stressed or angry patients, reduce hypertension, improve outcomes from strokes and heart attacks, and help people sleep.

- Watch Leo Buscaglia on YouTube. He has passed, but his work will never die. Read his book *Love*. It is 99 cents on Amazon and one of the best books I have ever read.

- Challenge yourself to read Og Mandino's *The Greatest Salesman in the World*, which contains The Legend of the 10 Scrolls, or commit to just one month of reading Scroll II: "I will greet this day with love in my heart."

- Support the heart chakra through meditations and breathing exercises.

- Use essential oils that will help balance out the heart chakra like rosewood or rose essence, which also can help clear repressed emotions and grief.

- Heart Meridian points are located on the body. It is great to practice these acupuncture points to help you and other people feel more relaxed. K27 is below the collar bone close to the sternum. Locate the C17 point, which is in the center of the sternum or breast-bone. This area helps the overall flow in the body. Find H7, which is located on the wrist palm side up directly linear to the pinky on the wrist. It is recommended to rub or apply light pressure to these areas for one minute and do the breath work.

- An appropriate time to apply some of these techniques in a hospital setting is when the patient is on a heart monitor. We instruct them to use the diaphragmatic breathing exercise and watch the monitor for changes in heart rate. We have all seen the heart rate increase with position changes and stress in the room. This is the other side of that spectrum. Remember, as high as 90% of illness and disease can be related to stress.

- There are many products on Amazon that can help with home monitoring and biofeedback. I bought my husband the Muse headband to teach him how to meditate. It is capable of monitoring your brain waves. It works great with meditation. As you meditate, it tells you whether or not you are in a relaxed state and helps you refocus when you are not. This can be a great supplement to (or replacement for) medications and counseling.

Music to Stimulate Both Sides of the Brain: Music therapy also shows efficacy in decreasing anxiety levels and improving functioning of depressed individuals.[34]

Reflexology: [35] Reflexology is about energy and energy blockages. There are simple pressure points to help us and our clients reduce anxiety and stress, including:

1. Hall of Impression point: located between the eyebrows. Simply rub or massage the area to relieve anxiety and stress.
2. Heavenly Gate point: located on your ear in the center of the upper ear. This area helps relieve insomnia, anxiety, and stress.
3. Shoulder well point: your shoulder muscle. This area relieves stress, reduce muscle tension and headaches.

4. Union Valley point: located on your hand between the thumb and the index finger.

5. Great Surge point: located on your foot three finger widths below the Intersection of your big toe and second toe. Helps relieve anxiety, stress, pain and menstrual cramps.

6. Inner Frontier Gate point: located on the wrist three finger widths away from the hand in between the tendon in the middle; do this palm facing up.

Shut Up and Redirect: Tell your brain to shut up. Redirect your thoughts. Think of a time in your life that you were happy and successful. Concentrate on that. Use this with patients. Have them concentrate on the times that they felt healthy and what that felt like.

The Thymus Thump: The thymus gland lies beneath the upper portion of the breastbone or sternum. The thymus is considered to be our happiness center. Activate your life energy and improve your mood by rubbing or thumping the thymus area. Thump or rub for 15 seconds or really breathe into it for 2 minutes. Bye bye stress and anxiety! Teach patients to thump while you are charting.

Visualization: When you think about tomorrow, you must think a new thought. Live on purpose! Imagine a life filled with beauty. Visualize and imprint on your brain what you want to have happen today. Be visually specific about what you are wearing, your mood, your location. Create the whole image, then utilize questions to help stimulate your brain to find another way of thinking and living, another solution. Author Noah St. John says, "If we ask better questions, our brain will look for better answers." It can be challenging to ask such questions as, "Why do I have so many gifts to share with the world? Why am I the best group facilitator in the world? Why do I have a bestseller?" These positive affirmations can feel arrogant, but they are the opposite. They inspire confidence and move us away from all of those "I can't" thoughts. Think of questions or visualization techniques you can encourage your patients to use while you are doing painful procedures. Whatever techniques you use, memorize them so they are always handy. [36]

Endnotes

1   https://www.ncbi.nlm.nih.gov/pmc/articles/PMC3037121/

2   https://www.heartmath.com/

3   https://www.hrdive.com/news/study-burnout-is-a-major-threat-to-employee-engagement

4   https://www.youtube.com/watch?v=oQ5_9dzqNNs

5   https://thework.com/instruction-the-work-byron-katie/

6   https://archive.org/details/JoseSilvaTheSilvaMindControlMethod/Jose-Silva--The-Silva-Mind-Control-?view=theater

7   https://www.makeuseof.com/tag/mind-mapping-sites-apps-brainstorm-ideas/

8   https://www.virtuesforlife.com/two-wolves/

9   https://www.ncbi.nlm.nih.gov/pmc/articles/PMC4286362/

10 https://www.sciencedirect.com/science/article/pii/S0091305703000443

11 https://psycnet.apa.org/record/2007-03392-002

12 https://journals.physiology.org/doi/full/10.1152/jappl.2000.88.2.774

13 https://www.purewow.com/wellness/energy-work

14 https://www.selfhelppod.com/what-is-the-difference-between-meridians-and-chakras-how-to-

15 https://www.counseling.org/news/aca-blogs/aca-member-blogs/aca-member-blogs/2019/05/20/acupressure-meridians-and-tapping

16 https://www.healthline.com/nealth/eft-tapping

17 https://www.seattlechildrens.org/pdf/PE2256.pdf

18 https://academic.oup.com/cercor/article/29/6/2331/5017785

19 https://www.masterco.org

20 https://birminghamclinicalhypnotherapy.com/brain-waves-and-

trance/

21 https://www.nccih.nih.gov/health/meditation-in-depth.

22 https://www.sciencedirect.com/science/article/abs/pii/
S0965229918312913

23 https://www.theatlantic.com/health/archive/2014/07/people-pre-
fer-electric-shocks-to-being-alone-with-their-thoughts/373936/

24 https://www.stylecraze.com/articles/types-brain-waves-ef-
fects-meditation/

25 https://www.ahajournals.org/doi/full/10.1161/CIRCOUT-
COMES.112.967406

26 https://www.ncbi.nlm.nih.gov/pmc/articles/PMC5866112/

27 S.T.O.P Is a Mindfulness Trick to Calm You Down | The Muse

28 Six mindfulness techniques for physicians (medicalnewstoday.
com)

29 https://www.businessinsider.com/only-7-seconds-to-make-first-
impression-2013-4

30 Narrative Medicine: the Importance of Storytelling in Health Care
| For Better | US News

31 https://storybrand.com

32 https://healthyinteractions.com/conversation-map-tools

33 https://www.ncbi.nlm.nih.gov/pmc/articles/PMC539473/

34 These 6 Types of Music Are Known to Dramatically Improve Productivity (entrepreneur.com)

35 https://www.healthline.com/health/pressure-points-for-anxi-
ety#inner-frontier-gate

36 3 Effective Visualization Techniques to Change Your Life | Psy-
chology Today

About the Author

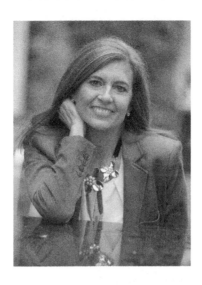

Donna C. Naumann has been a nationally certified Family Nurse Practitioner since 2002. She has completed studies in Functional Medicine, Reiki, Pranic Healing, Hypnosis, Neuro Linguistics Programming and Group Medical Visits with hundreds of hours practicing in all health modalities. Mrs. Naumann owned a family medical practice that created, for her an environment of stress and long hours that frequently demanded working nights and weekends. Learning how to balance life and create energy and promote health became her obsession. She gained interest in alternative health solutions through her years of experience with her patients who never overcame disease, just managed it. As she, herself healed she began to teach her patients that their stress levels, eating patterns, and energy levels needed to be better handled to create longevity and a structure of coping with life's multiple levels of stress internally and externally. Food as medicine, meditation as a solution base to stress as well as the numerous tips she shares in this book will help us all stay present and learn to take care of ourselves and teach others to do the same.

Made in the USA
Monee, IL
18 August 2022

11460735R00105